Conception, Pregnancy and Birth

Edited by

Catherine A. Niven RGN, BSc, PhD
Reader in Psychology
Glasgow Caledonian University

and

Anne Walker BSc, PhD
Lecturer in Health Psychology
University of Leeds

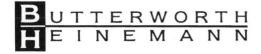

Butterworth-Heinemann
Linacre House, Jordan Hill, Oxford OX2 8DP
A division of Reed Educational & Professional Publishing Ltd

A member of the Reed Elsevier plc group

OXFORD   BOSTON   JOHANNESBURG
MELBOURNE   NEW DELHI   SINGAPORE

First published 1996

© Reed Educational & Professional Publishing 1996

British Library Cataloguing in Publication Data

A catalogue record for this book is available from the British Library

Library of Congress Cataloguing in Publication Data

A catalogue record for this book is available from the Library of Congress

ISBN 0 7506 2250 4

Typeset by EJS Chemical Composition, Midsomer Norton, Bath
Printed and bound by Hartnolls Ltd, Bodmin, Cornwall

The Psychology of Reproduction 2

Conception, Pregnancy and Birth

Contents

Series preface

Sex, gender, adolescence, menstruation, pregnancy, childbirth, parenthood – these experiences are linked by their relationship to human reproduction. Reproductive experiences and behaviours can be divided into four broad categories. First, there are those concerned with the activity of reproduction: pregnancy and childbirth, for instance. Second are those to do with the potential for reproduction: puberty, menstruation and the menopause, for example. Going through puberty or having menstrual periods does not in itself constitute reproduction, but people who do not experience these things usually are not able to experience active reproduction either. What might be considered the prototypical reproductive activity, heterosexual sexual intercourse, does not fit neatly into either of these categories. In the late twentieth century, and perhaps for many centuries, only a minority of sexual acts are concerned with reproduction. The creation of another human being is only one of the many reasons for engaging in sexual activity of whatever type, so sex might be better considered as an activity with reproductive potential, rather than a reproductive act. A third category of activities and experiences are those concerned with fertility control: the things we do and decisions we make to control whether or not we have children, and a fourth category is concerned with the consequences of reproductive activity: prenatal development, parenthood and parent–child relationships. These four elements of reproduction form a large part of many people's lives.

Reproduction is fundamental to human life. If we were all to decide tomorrow not to reproduce, then there would simply be no more people. How often we reproduce has economic and social implications for all areas of a society. The effects of the post-war 'baby boom' on education policy, employment possibilities and the care of older people can be clearly seen in our own society, for example. On a more global scale, the human population explosion has devastating environmental effects and significant qualitative costs for those humans who are produced, in terms of inadequacy of resources. Most governments attempt to control the reproductive activity of their people – either discouraging or limiting reproduction in a variety of ways, or promoting reproduction for religious or political reasons (Fathalla, 1992). Restrictive methods of control may range from the provision of family planning services and the discouragement of parenthood outside marriage to enforced sterilization programmes. Governments may encourage (or enforce) parenthood by not providing contraceptive information and/or access to abortion, by not educating women or encouraging women to be economically independent (hence promoting motherhood as the only choice). Clearly, reproduction is important for societies.

Reproduction is also a concern for individuals. Most people will have children at some time in their lives and are concerned about when to conceive children and how many children to have. Individuals, like governments, may be influenced by political, religious or economic factors in the desire to have children or remain child-free. Other more individual factors are involved though, such as a sense of identity as a parent, a need for 'immortality', pressure from potential grandparents, a desire to consolidate a relationship or a wish to be closely involved with a child from its earliest moments (see Walker and McNeill, 1991). Our society clearly sees the ability and desire to have children as 'normal' – writers in newspapers and magazines express sympathy for people who are unable to have children, and many pounds and dollars are spent on technologies to assist conception for the involuntarily childless. Choosing to remain childfree, by contrast, is less likely to be viewed positively, and women especially who decide not to have children may be seen as 'selfish' or 'unnatural' (Matlin, 1993).

Societies and cultures have not only controlled how many children people may have, but also the circumstances in which children may be conceived (e.g. only within marriage) and in which they are born (e.g. in hospital). In the late twentieth century control of conception has extended from the ability to prevent pregnancy (which has always been practised to some extent), to the ability, through technology, to enable conception in circumstances which would previously have prevented it. At present, the technology is far from perfect and many people who attempt to conceive using the new reproductive technologies are disappointed. However, the capacity for control both of conception and of gestation are present, with alarming moral and ethical implications, especially for women (Rowland, 1992; Chadwick, 1992).

Pictures of parents holding a longed-for baby whose conception was only possible through modern technology are emotive and heart-warming. Few of us could fail to be moved by them. They imply though that reproduction is a purely mechanical process, involving only the chance, or planned, meeting of sperm and egg. Of course, the physiological and mechanical processes involved in becoming pregnant, sustaining pregnancy and giving birth are important if we want to understand human reproduction. But as we have seen, reproduction has meaning both for individual men and women, and for society. Reproduction is not just a physical event. It also has psychological and social implications.

So, what is the 'psychology of reproduction'? From its earliest beginnings, psychologists have concerned themselves with some aspects of the reproductive process. Heterosexual sex and the development of gender identity have been of particular interest to researchers. Child development, both before and after birth, has also attracted attention. Few attempts have been made, however, to draw this research together as a coherent discipline. The establishment of the Society for Reproductive and Infant Psychology (SRIP) in the early 1980s, and its journal, the *Journal of Reproductive and Infant Psychology* (JRIP) in 1983, acknowledged the growth of psychological research in areas relating to reproduction, and the likely further growth in these areas resulting from the development of 'new reproductive technologies'. In the first editorial of the journal, Christopher Macy outlines the scope of reproductive and infant psychology as follows:

... pregnancy and infancy ... might be regarded as central concerns within the field of reproduction .... But in order to understand women's experience of pregnancy we need to understand why women become pregnant .... We must look at the social value systems surrounding childbearing and childrearing, and equally at the psychological parameters associated with childlessness and infertility .... We take the view that psychological aspects of contraception and termination also fall squarely in our field as do many aspects of the psychology of women.

We would add to this by suggesting that many aspects of the 'psychology of men' fall into the remit of reproductive psychology too. The cultural tendency to see reproduction as 'women's work' has resulted in a neglect of men's experiences of puberty, fertility, contraception, sexuality, fatherhood and so on. The emphasis on women in this series of books should not be taken to imply that we consider reproduction only to be women's concern.

Reproductive issues have been approached from a variety of perspectives within psychology. The chief areas of interest have lain within clinical psychology and developmental psychology. Hence, the research which falls into the scope of reproductive psychology is dominated by 'problem-focused' studies and/or studies of infants and small children, rather than investigations of normative experiences. Not surprisingly, there is more to be said about reproductive activities and consequences than there is about reproductive potential and fertility control. Reproductive issues have attracted interest from a variety of other disciplines and epistemological movements too, which have influenced the approach of psychologists. The largest influence is that of the biomedical sciences. Since psychology has adopted similar research methods, and has often been concerned with similar research questions, biomedical themes have had a significant impact. This impact is shown in the concern of psychologists with psychiatric indices and labels of distress (e.g. post-natal depression) or with the psychological factors which predict distress, rather than understanding the experiences of people who are not distressed. Some psychologists have made important steps towards redressing this imbalance, however. For example, Myra Hunter's longitudinal studies of women going through the menopause (see Chapter 4 of Volume 1) have challenged the assumption from clinical studies that the menopause is necessarily a time of emotional turmoil and psychological dysfunction.

In addition to an emphasis on 'problems' such as post-natal depression, infertility, etc., the biomedical influence has also endorsed a positivist, hypothesis-testing approach within psychology. This approach usually requires measurement of experiences, and psychologists have played a role in developing a number of inventories and tools for quantifying distress or psychological state. Scores on such measures can be correlated with other factors in epidemiological surveys or used to evaluate interventions in treatment trials. Randomized controlled trials and measurement of experiences are clearly important in the appropriate context. However, the exclusivity of this approach in psychology has been criticized (e.g. Hollway, 1989; Potter and Wetherell, 1987). The emphasis on the use of existing measures can reduce the sensitivity of research to the specific experiences of participants in a particular study, and assumes that the quantification of experiences such as depression, joy, anxiety or pain is meaningful as well as functional. For these reasons, many researchers are turning towards qualitative or postmodernist approaches within psychology. In addition, a hypothesis-testing approach can encourage reductionism, that is the tendency to see the factor evaluated as the only important one. For example, if we test the hypothesis that anxiety management techniques reduce the intensity of pain during labour, and find them to be effective, then we (or others) may be tempted to infer that anxiety is the only important factor in labour pain. Clearly in this case that is a ridiculous conclusion. In other circumstances, though, the involvement of multiple factors may not be so apparent. The inadequacy of single-factor biomedical models to explain many modern health-related experiences has resulted in the development of biopsychosocial approaches to health and illness (e.g. Engel, 1977) and the birth of the new sub-discipline of health psychology. A biopsychosocial influence can be seen clearly in many of the chapters of this series, with reproductive psychologists avoiding reductionism by explicitly placing their work within a multi-factored framework (e.g. Ussher, 1992; Hunter, 1994). The influence of the biomedical approach and its emphasis on problems, quantification and reductionism will also be seen throughout this series.

A second influence is feminism and feminist theory. As we have already said, reproduction has historically been seen as the defining characteristic of womankind. The view of woman as a womb-container has had profound implications as many feminist writers have pointed out (e.g. Martin, 1989; Ussher, 1989). To attribute experiences such as premenstrual syndrome, post-natal depression, depression in middle age, emotionality in pregnancy, and so on, simply to the biological or psychological consequences of the female reproductive system is to ignore the effects of a patriarchal culture on women. Many feminist writers have described the inherent gender bias in modern societies which influences women's positions within heterosexual relationships, our earning capacity and the expectations held about the unpaid work we will do (e.g. Oakley, 1993). Women on average are poorer than men, whether employed or not. Women are more likely to be the recipients of domestic violence and sexual abuse. Women are more likely to care for children, ageing relatives or other dependent family members. In these circumstances it is at best misogynist to attribute distress solely to biological circumstances, or to attempt to adapt women's biology to enable us to cope with intolerable situations. So, feminist critiques are demanding the contextualization of women's reproductive experiences. A further impact of feminism in social science has been the questioning of power relationships within the research process and the critique of science itself as a patriarchal institution (see Harding, 1991). Medicine has been deconstructed as an instrument of social control – especially of women (see Ehrenreich and English, 1978; Showalter, 1987). Psychology too can be a powerful social control mechanism. The implications of this critique for the processes of doing research and reporting findings are far reaching. The interpretation of research as a political activity raises questions about who is doing the research, why they are doing it, who is paying for it and what the perceived benefits are. Many feminists are struggling to develop research methodologies which do not reinforce the imbalance of power between 'researcher' and 'researched', and which offer benefits for research participants in terms of empowerment, for example (see Neilson, 1990). These approaches have as yet had little influence on mainstream psychology, but the concern of reproductive psychology with the psychology of women means that they are having more of an impact here.

The purpose of this series of three books is to bring together the disparate strands of research and theory which can be called reproductive psychology. In our own work with undergraduate psychology, nursing and midwifery students, we have often felt the need for a single source of reference which could allow students to see the breadth and scope of psychological approaches to human reproduction. Our original intention was to bring these together in a single volume. The number of topics to be covered and the vigour of current research activity surprised us though, and we soon realized that a single volume would be inadequate to encompass it all. So, we have solicited contributions from currently active researchers for a three-volume series. The subject matter of each volume reflects the categories within reproductive psychology which we outlined at the beginning of this introduction. The first volume is concerned with reproductive potential and fertility control, the second with reproductive activity – conception, pregnancy and birth – and the third with the consequences of reproduction – early development, parenting and so on. There is no particular beginning or end to this series, although we have arranged the contributions in what seems to us to be a logical order. The circularity of human reproduction is apparent though; once the child has been born then she or he begins the process of gender identity and the development of their own reproductive potential, and so on. Like the seasons of the year, reproduction has no particular beginning or end. It is a continuous process, influencing all of our lives whether we are reproductively active or not. We hope that, like us, you will find the psychology of human reproduction, despite its inadequacies and omissions, a fascinating topic and that you will learn something of personal as well as academic interest from these books.

Anne Walker
Catherine A. Niven
1995

References

Chadwick, R. (ed.) (1992). *Ethics, Reproduction and Genetic Control.* Revised edn. London: Routledge.

Ehrenreich, B. and English, E. (1978). *For Her Own Good: A Hundred Years of Experts' Advice to Women.* New York: Anchor Doubleday.

Engel, G. L. (1977). The need for a new medical model. *Science,* **196**, 129–36.

Fathalla, M. F. (1992). Society and reproductive life. In *Reproductive Life: Advances in Psychosomatic Obstetrics and Gynaecology* (K. Wijma and B. von Schoultz, eds). Carnforth: Parthenon.

Harding, S. (1991). *Whose Science? Whose Knowledge?* Milton Keynes: Open University Press.

Hollway, W. (1989). *Subjectivity and Method in Psychology: Gender, Meaning and Science.* London: Sage.

Hunter, M. (1994). *Counselling in Obstetrics and Gynaecology.* Leicester: BPS Books.

Macy, C. (1983). The Society for Reproductive and Infant Psychology: a statement of aims. *Journal of Reproductive and Infant Psychology,* **1** (1) 1–4.

Martin, E. (1989). *The Woman in the Body.* Milton Keynes: Open University Press.

Matlin, M. (1993). *The Psychology of Women.* 2nd edn. New York: Harcourt Brace Jovanovich.

Nielson, J. M. (ed.) (1990). *Feminist Research Methods.* Boulder, CO: Westview Press.

Oakley, A. (1993). *Essays on Women, Medicine and Health.* Edinburgh: Edinburgh University Press.

Potter, J. and Wetherell, M. (1987). *Discourse and Social Psychology*. London: Sage.

Rowland, R. (1992). *Living Laboratories: Women and Reproductive Technology*. London: Lime Tree.

Showalter, E. (1987). *The Female Malady*. London: Virago.

Ussher, J. (1989). *The Psychology of the Female Body*. London: Routledge.

Ussher, J. (1992). Research and theory related to female reproduction: Implications for clinical psychology. *British Journal of Clinical Psychology*, **31**, 129–51.

Walker, A. and McNeill, E. (eds) (1991). Family planning and reproductive decisions. *Journal of Reproductive and Infant Psychology*, Theme Issue, **9** (4).

Preface to Volume 2

This volume introduces its themes through a chapter on reproductive decision-making; the necessary first step in the reproductive process. Chapters 2 and 3 recognize that the decision to reproduce may not always be followed by conception but that a variety of techniques are now available to help couples in this situation. Chapter 4 deals with pregnancy from the perspective of the mother, and Chapter 5 from the perspective of the fetus, and as such these chapters set the scene for the remainder of the book which deals with events which may follow conception: prenatal screening in Chapter 6, antenatal preparation in Chapter 8 and the variety of birth experiences discussed in Chapters 9 and 10. Chapters 7 and 12 discuss pregnancies which sadly do not end in live births. Chapter 11 deals with one perhaps unwelcome consequence of reproduction – pain – illustrating how admirably people cope with this and other aspects of the reproductive process. Despite having been involved in reproductive research for many years, it is this ability to cope which strikes us anew when we contemplate the numerous difficulties associated with reproduction which beset mothers, fathers, families and fetuses.

It seems useful to draw the reader's attention to the robustness of the human organism since psychology texts of this sort tend to focus on problems and difficulties. Yet arguably in reproductive psychology, more that in any other area of psychology, there is ample scope for examining achievement and joy.

As we stated in the Series preface, it has been our intention to examine the events associated with reproduction from a bio-psycho-social perspective. In doing this we are placing the series within a framework currently in the ascendancy in health psychology. However, a recurring theme within this volume is that the psychological literature related to childbirth and the events surrounding it has developed in isolation from other areas in health psychology and has remained uninformed by many of the theories, concepts and treatment approaches which are currently influential in health psychology, e.g. by theories such as self-efficacy theory or cognitive appraisal and in treatment approaches involving debriefing following traumatic stress or the psychological management of pain. This book goes a long way towards correcting these deficiencies.

Research into the psychological aspects of pregnancy and birth suffers from a number of methodological problems involving small sample sizes, non-representative samples, and a lack of control groups. These problems reflect ethical and practical difficulties which are inherent in research of this kind. In pregnancy and birth, ethical considerations extend to the fetus/baby as well as to the mother and these 'secondary subjects' are of course in no position to grant consent to research participation, informed or otherwise. Thus many ethics committees automatically rule out routine research in pregnancy, only allowing research which has clear benefit for the participants and carries no risk at all to the fetus. This constrains the type of research which can be carried out and affects funding, leading to a plethora of 'problem-centred' research.

Access to subjects in pregnancy is difficult since pregnancy, unlike birth is not recorded publicly. Thus access is usually through hospital or GP records or through groups which prepare women for childbirth such as the National Childbirth Trust. Thus many studies utilize subject groups attending hospital clinics or antenatal classes, consequently missing non-attenders and under-representing the younger, less educated and less socially advantaged section of the population who are less likely to attend antenatal classes.

During birth, access to a totally representative group of women in labour is theoretically possible since the vast majority of parturants give birth in hospital. However, many hospitals especially those in big cities, cater for a section of the population, often stratified in relation to economic circumstances. Thus research which is based in a single hospital may only tap the well-off or the more 'deprived' citizens of the city or (particularly in the US) may reflect the hospital's status as private or public.

Birth research suffers massive practical difficulties. The timing and duration of the event is unpredictable and frequently takes place in unsocial hours. If the subject is suffering labour pain, any interview or questionnaire will be constantly interrupted and the effects of pain-killing drugs may affect both the ability to respond and the quality of the response if obtainable. Delivery involves the baby in the most dangerous journey of its entire life. Safe delivery depends to a considerable extent on the expulsive efforts of the mother. Thus many people regard it as intrinsically unethical to do anything during delivery which might distract her from these efforts, such as administer a questionnaire. Many mothers are anyhow unable or unwilling to participate in any extraneous activity at this time.

The early postnatal period used to be a time when much data could be gathered since mothers were typically in hospital for about a week following delivery and were thus something of a captive audience for researchers. However, health policy changes towards 'patient' choice and care in the community now mean that many mothers and babies go home after 4–48 hours, leaving little time for participating in research in between recovering from the birth and getting to know the new baby.

All in all, a catalogue of challenge faces researchers in this field and the rich data they collect, which forms the basis of every chapter in this book, pays tribute to their patience, intelligence and sensitivity.

Catherine A. Niven
Anne Walker
1995

Acknowledgements

The existence of these books owes a great deal to the Society for Reproductive and Infant Psychology. Most of the authors are members of SRIP, and it is through the activities of the Society that we have become aware of their work. At a more personal level, SRIP has enabled both of us to develop our research interests and discuss our research findings in a supportive and friendly atmosphere. Many SRIP members, past and present, have influenced our thinking and encouraged us to continue to work in this area. Particular thanks are due to the founder members of the Society, and editors of the *Journal of Reproductive and Infant Psychology*, whose vision and commitment have made the editing of these books possible.

Thanks are also due to the authors of these chapters who responded to our editorial demands with good humour and speed and to Susan Devlin and Deborah Humphries at Butterworth-Heinemann for their patience and efficiency.

Contributors

Rosanne Cecil, BA, MSc, DPhil, Research Fellow
Rosanne Cecil is a Social Anthropologist at the Queen's University of Belfast. Her current research is in the field of miscarriage and other aspects of women's reproductive health. She has conducted research into a number of anthropological and sociological issues in the area of health and welfare. She is co-author (with J. Offer and F. St. Leger) of *Informal Welfare: A Sociological Study of Care in Northern Ireland* (Gower, 1987) and editor of *The Anthropology of Pregnancy Loss: Comparative Studies in Miscarriage, Stillbirth and Neonatal Death* (Berg, 1996).

Kevin Connolly, BSc, PhD, FBPsS
Kevin Connolly is Professor of Psychology at Sheffield University. He has been President of the British Psychological Society, Chairman of the Association of Child Psychology and Psychiatry and President of the Psychology Section of the British Association for the Advancement of Science. His research interests include the genetics and evolution of behaviour, most recently this has involved collaboration with geneticists in Chile. He has a long-standing interest in the development of motor skills and over the last fifteen years has worked on problems of malnutrition and parasitic disease in relation to the development of children. This work has involved studies in Papua New Guinea and Southern Africa. He is married, has three grown-up daughters and two grandchildren.

Robert Edelmann, BSc, MSc, MPhil, PhD
Robert Edelmann graduated from Birkbeck College, London, where he obtained his PhD in Psychology, and trained in Clinical Psychology at the Institute of Psychiatry, London. He has worked as a Lecturer in Psychology at the University of Sheffield and is currently a Senior Lecturer in Clinical Psychology at the University of Surrey. He is director of an MSc in Health Psychology and acting co-director of a Psych D in Clinical Psychology. His current research interests include social phobia and psychological aspects of infertility and the reproduction technologies. He is author of four books and over eighty book chapters and journal articles.

Josephine Emery, BSc(Hons), MSc, PhD
Having read physiology at Birmingham University, Josephine Emery worked for the Medical Research Council until marriage and family led to a career break. In the 1980s she gained a BSc(Hons) in Psychology and an MSc in Clinical Psychology from Manchester University. After experience in various teaching

hospitals in the north-west, Josephine took up a research post in the IVF unit at St Mary's Hospital in Manchester where she completed her PhD. She is currently working as a consultant in private practice based at the Alexandra Hospital in Cheadle with particular interests in medical and neurological psychology.

Karel Gijsbers, PhD

Karel Gijsbers is a Lecturer in Psychology at Stirling University contributing to courses in neuroscience and health psychology. Recent publications include studies of the effects on the brain of steroids released during stress, sex differences in the perception of experimental and clinical pain, and the use of pain-coping strategies by women giving birth. His current research is concerned with the origins and effectiveness of pain-coping strategies used spontaneously by athletes in training and women in labour.

Peter G. Hepper, BSc, PhD

Peter Hepper is currently Professor of Psychology at Queen's University and Director of the Fetal Behaviour Research Centre sponsored by the Wellcome Trust. He completed his undergraduate degree in Psychology at Exeter University before obtaining his PhD from Durham University. His research interests include all areas of fetal behaviour and neurological development.

Jenny Hewison, PhD

Jenny Hewison is a Senior Lecturer in Psychology at Leeds University. Currently, she is partly seconded to the Institute of Epidemiology and Health Services Research in Leeds, to do maternity services research. She also does work on health outcomes, on quality of life in chronic illness, and on factors influencing the health and development of children. She has more general research interests in psychological measurement, in methodology and statistics, and in the evaluation of interventions in applied settings. On a more personal note, but highly relevant to the psychology of reproduction, she is the mother of two young daughters.

Edith Hillan, PhD, MSc, DipLSc, RGN, RSCN, RM

Edith Hillan is a Senior Lecturer in the Department of Nursing and Midwifery Studies at the University of Glasgow. Having completed a graduate course in nursing, she then undertook further training in paediatrics and midwifery. After a period working in a Palestinian hospital she returned to the UK and midwifery practice as a labour ward sister in Glasgow Royal Maternity Hospital. Her research interests and publications include techniques of cervical ripening, a comparison of methods for labour induction, a randomized study of a birthing chair versus the dorsal recumbent position for delivery and the use of information technology in health care delivery. Her PhD thesis explored the physical and psychosocial outcomes of caesarean section in Glasgow. She is a member of the Research Advisory Committee of the Royal College of Obstetricians and Gynaecologists which amongst other activities distributes moneys raised by *Wellbeing* (formerly *Birthright*) for research.

Jane Littlewood, BSc, PhD

Jane Littlewood is a Senior Lecturer in Social Policy and Administration at Goldsmiths' College, University of London. Her major research area is concerned with women and loss and she is one of the co-founders of the Women and Welfare Research Group. Her recent publications include: *Aspects of Grief* (1992) Routledge; *Applied Research for Better Practice* (with A. Everitt, P. Hardiker and A. Mullender 1992) Macmillan; *'Widows Weeds and Women's Needs'* in Wilkinson, S. and Kitzinger, C. (Eds.) *Women and Health: Feminist Perspectives* (1994) Taylor-Francis and *The Myth of Madonna: Postnatal Depression and Maternal Distress* (with N. McHugh, in press) Macmillan.

Catherine Niven, RGN, BSc, PhD
Catherine Niven is Reader in Psychology at Glasgow University. She is well known for her work in reproductive psychology being the author of *Psychological Care for Families* published by Butterworth-Heinemann in 1992 and editor with Douglas Carroll of *Health Psychology of Women* published by Harwood Academic Publications. Her current research is in the area of health and reproduction with special focus on the well-being of premature babies and the study of pain in childbirth.

Lyn Quine, BA(Hons), PhD
Dr Lyn Quine is a health psychologist who has worked at the University of Kent for fifteen years. She has a joint appointment as Senior Research Fellow with the University and South Kent Community Healthcare NHS Trust. She has published in a variety of health psychology and medical journals and has jointly authored two books on health psychology. Her main research interests lie in maternal and child health, and she has a particular interest in psychosocial and behavioural factors affecting pregnancy outcome.

Derek Rutter, PhD
Dr Derek Rutter is Reader in Social Psychology at the University of Kent. His main research is in health, and he has published widely on social psychological predictors of health outcomes. Recent projects have focused on pregnancy outcome and infant well-being, breast cancer screening, and motorcycling safety. He is co-author of *Social Psychological Approaches to Health*, published by Harvester Wheatsheaf in 1993.

Gill Scott, BSc Econ (Sociology)
Gill Scott is a Senior Lecturer in Sociology in the Department of Social Sciences at Glasgow Caledonian University. She has been involved in teaching and working with health professionals for over fifteen years. Her previous publications include various articles and reports on aspects of mothers and social policy. Current research interests include the social factors affecting families with young children in Scotland and the changing pattern of resources available to women combining work and parenting.

Pauline Slade, BSc, MSc, PhD, CPsychol
Pauline Slade is Senior Lecturer in Clinical Psychology at University of Sheffield and Consultant Clinical Psychologist. She has worked in the field of reproductive psychology for over 20 years both in terms of her research and her clinical work. She has published extensively in this field, in particular, on

psychological aspects of menstrual cycle and menopausal problems, infertility, experiences of labour and the post partum and non continuing pregnancies.

Anne Woollett, BA, PhD
Anne Woollett is Reader in the Department of Psychology, University of East London. Her research interests are in areas of women's reproductive health, including pregnancy, childbirth, reproductive decision making, mothering and motherhood, and the development of children and young people. With Paula Nicolson from University of Sheffield and Harriette Marshall from University of Staffordshire she is currently researching the ideas and experiences of mothers from a range of ethnic backgrounds living in East London. With Ann Phoenix and Eva Lloyd she co-edited *Motherhood: Meanings, Practices and Ideologies* (Sage, 1991) and with David White wrote *Families as a Context for Development* (The Falmer Press, 1992).

Reproductive decisions

Anne Woollett

In the opening chapter of this book, Anne Woollett examines the first stage in the process of reproduction – the decision to reproduce – one over which women now have more control than at any time in the past. Despite this, as the author shows, the processes underlying reproductive decisions have been poorly understood. Until recently, we probably knew more about why people chose one particular brand of jeans than why they chose to have, or not have a baby. However, current research is addressing vital issues in this regard, revealing the psychological mechanisms which drive reproductive decisions, the ways in which men's and women's decision-making varies, and the social and economic pressures which can have a powerful influence on the nature and timing of such decisions.

This chapter follows on from chapters in Volume 1 of this series which deal with gender identity, contraception, sexuality and sexual behaviour.

Introduction

In this chapter I will consider some of the many decisions people make about reproduction, the ideas they draw upon when making their choices and the ways in which psychologists and others have explained these decisions. People's ideas and choices about reproduction and about themselves as parents are seen as private and personal concerns. But they are made in an ideological and cultural context which both reflects and shapes people's reproductive decisions. This includes ideas prevalent in a culture about children and families and about women and men's roles and their identities as adults. Because contraception, pregnancy, childbirth and parenting impact more directly on women's lives and identities than on men's, women's reproductive decisions have been more thoroughly investigated. The ability of men and women to translate their aspirations and choices into action is increasingly linked to their access to reproductive technologies, such as contraception and abortion to prevent or delay pregnancy, and more recently to infertility treatment to assist conception.

Why people want children

A number of explanations of people's ideas and choices about having children and becoming parents have been proposed. Sociobiology accounts consider that the desire for children is based on 'instincts' and especially on women's 'maternal instincts' whereas men's desire for parenthood is more often viewed in terms of ensuring the survival of their genes. In contrast, economic models view reproductive decision-making as a more complex process balancing the costs and benefits of children (Michaels, 1988). The economic costs and benefits of parenting vary from culture to culture and from group to group within a culture, and depend on factors such as the contribution children make to the family economy and the costs children incur for parents through childcare, education and constraints on maternal employment opportunities.

Most research about why people want children has been conducted in the developed world and concentrates on the psychological and social impact of having children rather than on the economic costs or the physical risks for women and children. These psychological costs include the disapproval of family and others of parenting in 'wrong' situations, for example, as single parents, the psychological costs associated with childlessness for those who do not have children, and, as children grow older, loss of their income, support, and domestic work (Boulton, 1983; Busfield, 1974; Fawcett, 1988; Llewelyn and Osborne, 1990; Michaels, 1988; Sheeran, White and Phillips, 1991). This research indicates that children are seen as costly to bring up and often as restricting their parents' opportunities and activities. However, these costs are generally perceived to be outweighed by the status associated with parenting, and the personal and emotional satisfactions children bring.

The salience of particular values, benefits and costs depends on people's social and economic circumstances and on the ideological and cultural context in which they live. People's accounts of their reproductive 'decisions' can sometimes usefully be considered rational, but often they appear to be less straightforward, reflecting the ambivalence and complexity of their ideas as they balance differing and sometimes contradictory ideas and pressures (Michaels, 1988). So, for example, children are seen as providing fun and enjoyment and emotional satisfaction in spite of the physical and emotional costs of childcare. They enhance parents' status and give them opportunities for expressing and receiving affection and establishing close relationships. With their children women and men can develop relations which are closer and more intimate than is usually possible in a non-family setting (Boulton, 1983; Busfield, 1974; Woollett, 1991; Michaels, 1988; Newson and Newson, 1968).

Motherhood provides a structure for women's lives, giving them a clear role and social function and more autonomy and control than in many others areas of their lives. Motherhood may provide a validation of a woman's adult status and female identity and demonstrates her physical and psychological adequacy. Having children grants women entry into a world of female knowledge and experience, and a common sense of purpose and identity with other women. Motherhood is also seen as providing women with an opportunity for personal growth and development, enabling them to recapture the psychic fusion they experienced with their own mothers, and to experience unconditional love (Llewelyn and Osborne, 1990). The increased responsibility of parenthood is often viewed as making both men and women more mature (Antonis, 1981; Michaels, 1988; Woollett, 1991).

While these are benefits to which many people subscribe, women often also report losses and costs. These include the hard work of motherhood, loneliness and depression, especially when women live in isolated settings, and loss of identity as separate individuals. For women in nuclear families, motherhood is often associated with a return to traditional gender roles and less support and understanding from male partners (Oakley, 1981; Boulton, 1983; Croghan, 1991; Llewelyn and Osborne, 1990; New and David, 1985). While such losses are commonly reported in accounts of women's experiences of motherhood, they rarely feature in studies of the values of children or in accounts of reproductive decision-making. This reflects a discrepancy between ideological and cultural prescriptions for motherhood/parenthood and women's everyday experiences (Phoenix, Woollett and Lloyd, 1991).

Couple relationship: 'making a family'

Psychological accounts often stress the benefits of children for their parents' relationship. In many cultures, children are construed as 'bringing a couple together' and as an essential 'next step' in a relationship and sometimes as a way of strengthening a couple's links with their wider family networks. Children may be seen as a physical manifestation of their parents' relationship and evidence of the strength of each person's commitment to the relationship and to one another. There is, however, no evidence to suggest that children do have these effects nor that couples with children are less susceptible to divorce and family breakdown than those without (Woollett, 1991).

However, in cultures such as the USA and the UK, children are increasingly born to mothers who are unmarried and, as a result of high divorce rates, grow up in households without their fathers or with step-parents and stepbrothers and sisters. The desire for children and the popularity of motherhood/parenthood remains high even though ideas have changed about the value or necessity of marriage as the appropriate setting for child rearing and increasing variety in family forms (Busfield, 1974; Lees, 1993; Phoenix, 1990; Woollett, 1991).

Avoiding childlessness

Another reason for having children, in spite of their costs and the restrictions on parents' activities, is that children enable women and men to avoid childlessness which is stigmatized and negatively evaluated in all cultures. Those who choose not to have children are often seen as unnatural and selfish, and those with fertility problems as desperate and to be pitied. Whatever the reason for their childlessness, childless men and women (and especially women) are denied the means of achieving maturity and adult status. Instead they are seen as leading lives which are either barren and unfulfilled, or filled with meaningless and second rate activities (Campbell, 1985; Pfeffer and Woollett, 1983; Woollett, 1991; Mason, 1993; Franklin, 1989). The stigma associated with childlessness and the strong negative feelings directed towards childless people indicate just how much having children is construed as part of the 'natural order' of society in all cultures (Busfield, 1974).

Diversity in people's ideas

Psychological research demonstrates that most people want to have children and become parents but there is also evidence of considerable variability in people's ideas about parenthood and the value of children and in the ways in which people make reproductive decisions.

People's ideas about the financial costs and benefits of having children vary according to their social, family and economic circumstances, cultural expectations about children's contribution to the family economy and what it costs to bring up and educate children. Parents who are affluent can forgo children's economic contribution; they can provide them with the toys, activities and consumer durables which are seen as essential for children's care and development in much of the developed world, and can purchase childcare. Women who live in close-knit family networks may share the work of childcare and so have more opportunity to be economically active than is the case for women who have total responsibility for the care of their children. Women in full-time employment experience greater economic and social disruption when they become mothers than do women who are not employed outside the home. There has been little research on the impact of social and economic context, but such variations are likely to influence women's experiences of bringing up children and hence their decisions about when to have children or how many children to have (Fawcett, 1988).

Because women rather than men have been the main focus of research, less is known about men's ideas about families and their reproductive decisions. Those studies which have examined men's choices suggest that, like women, men consider parenthood as a normal and expected part of adult life, but there are some differences in emphasis (Owens, 1982; Mason, 1993). British and US studies suggest that men tend to talk more explicitly than women about the enjoyment they anticipate in having a child to play with and in watching them grow up, but they are not as likely to report that their lives would be unsatisfying and dull without children (Payne, 1978; Busfield, 1974). Men's disappointments around infertility are often expressed in terms of their disappointment at preventing their female partners becoming mothers (Owens, 1982), indicating that while children are important for men, they impact less directly on men's identities and everyday lives (Phoenix, Woollett and Lloyd, 1991). Little is known directly about the ways in which men and women negotiate their reproductive decisions, including decisions about contraceptive practice (Sheeran, White and Phillips, 1991). Evidence is derived mainly from women's accounts of their male partner's ideas and preferences, suggesting that women are aware of men's ideas especially when they differ from their own (Woollett, Dosanjh-Matwala and Hadlow, 1991).

In some cultures it is assumed that employment (especially full-time employment outside the home) is incompatible with motherhood, especially for women with young children. However many mothers are economically active and there is interest in the ways in which employment impacts upon their ideas about children, parenting and their family roles (Westwood and Bhachu, 1988). There are some suggestions that in western cultures women with 'careers' decide not to have children or to delay childbearing, but there is little evidence that for the majority of women a commitment to employment alters their commitment to parenting and/or their ideas about the value of children (Lewis, 1991). Nor is there evidence that mothers in the USA or in the UK who are committed to employment use different parenting strategies than do mothers with a lesser commitment to work (Greenberger and Goldberg, 1989; Lewis, 1991).

Parity also influences parents' reproductive decisions. People's motives for wanting second or subsequent children differ somewhat from those for wanting a first child. A first child changes a woman's (and a man's) status and identity, creates a family and meets many of the needs/values identified above. There is, however, a strong commitment to having a second child (and often subsequent children), but the motives parents give are somewhat different. These include wanting to have both male and female children and to experience the challenge of bringing up a child with a different personality, and for first-born children to have the companionship of a brother or sister (Daniels and Weingarten, 1982; Michaels, 1988).

Ideological and cultural contexts

Discussion of the reasons why parents want children indicates the extent to which having children is constructed as 'normal' and 'natural' and as an essential aspect of adult life for men and women (but especially for women) in spite of the financial and psychological costs. This view of the normality of parenting and the values of children provides a powerful ideological framework within which men and women make their reproductive decisions, as Busfield (1974) argues:

> A society or a social group's patterns of reproduction occurs in an ideological context where particular beliefs, both those about reproduction per se and others that have reproductive consequences, affect, and are affected by, that pattern of reproduction. These beliefs provide a cognitive framework which structures individual action: they constitute the social reality in which reproduction takes place and they offer guidelines for, and justifications of, the actions of members of a society, which in aggregate result in a particular level of fertility.

In the developed world ideas about the family as the 'normal' and indeed as the 'best' context for adults to gain emotional satisfaction as well as for children's development are central to the ideological framework which shapes people's choices and decisions (New and David, 1985; Phoenix and Woollett, 1991). This is in spite of substantial changes in the stability of families, in their composition and in expectations about how men and women fulfil their family roles. Young people are aware of these changes and they are reflected in the ambivalence they frequently express about marriage and having children. The majority of 15 year olds are committed to becoming parents but comments such as 'Not until I've sorted out my life' and 'I want to be free from ties' indicate that children are also seen as restricting and as preventing women from pursuing other goals (Calvert and Stanton, 1992; Lees, 1993; Woollett, 1992). However, most young people do later become parents, indicating the pervasiveness of the pronatalist ideology as well as a lack of acceptable alternatives. Reproductive decisions are, therefore, often not so much about 'whether to have children' but about 'when' or 'how many' or 'how to combine motherhood with other roles'.

This ideological context helps to explain why people find difficulty in articulating their reproductive decisions. When they behave in ways which are 'normal' and 'given', people rarely need to articulate or explain their ideas. For this reason research on reproductive decision-making often examines men and women who because their experiences are 'non-normative' (because of infertility or their choice not to have children) have had to consider and give accounts of their reasons for wanting or not wanting to become parents (Veevers, 1980; Woollett, 1991).

The variety of reproductive decisions

During the course of their reproductive lives people make a variety of decisions. These are complicated and include decisions about not becoming pregnant as well as becoming pregnant, about when to become pregnant, how many children to have, what means (if any) to employ to prevent or ensure a pregnancy, and how effectively to employ these techniques (Porter, 1991).

Avoiding pregnancy

The number of children to which women give birth is decreasing in almost all cultures and so major reproductive decisions for people in heterosexual relationships who are sexually active involve the decisions to avoid pregnancy and the means of doing so (Owens, 1982; Porter, 1991). Men's and women's choices about the ways to avoid pregnancy are influenced by the methods available, the costs of different methods and their preferences about those methods, including concerns about the impact of contraception on their health and fertility, and the acceptability of non-medical means of controlling fertility (such as late marriage or abstaining from sexual intercourse) (see Chapter 7 in Volume 1 for a fuller discussion of contraception and contraceptive choices). Because of the difficulties people experience in giving accounts of their decisions and the thinking which underlies them, the basis on which these decisions are made and the relationship between reproductive decisions and contraceptive use are not well understood (Porter, 1991; Hubert, 1974; Oakley, 1981; Sheeran, White and Phillips, 1991).

Deciding to have a child

Most men and women expect to have children and become parents at some point in their lives (Michaels, 1988; Phoenix, Woollett and Lloyd, 1991). Because they assume they will become mothers, decisions about women's education, training and employment are often made in terms of how they relate to motherhood (Lees, 1993; Lewis, 1991; Llewelyn and Osborne, 1990). The availability of contraception and safe abortion has changed women's (and men's) ability to control their fertility but have had little impact on the proportion of people who become or expect to become parents. Similarly economic conditions and changing ideas about women's involvement in the labour force, which mean that in many countries mothers with young children are now often in paid employment, have not influenced the numbers of women having children nor current ideology about the optimal conditions for bringing up children (Lewis, 1991; Phoenix and Woollett, 1991). These (and other) changes have influenced the numbers of children women have, the age at which women have a first child and how they combine motherhood with employment, but have not changed expectations about motherhood and the proportion of women who become mothers.

Deciding to have a first child

The ideology around parenting also relates to the timing of a first birth and the circumstances in which women have children (Busfield, 1974). In many countries, it was expected that only those who were married would have children and premarital conceptions were quickly followed by marriage. In many developed societies, motherhood without marriage or even without cohabitation is now more readily accepted. It is often considered that a short delay between marriage and the birth of a first child is optimal to allow couples to 'set themselves up', 'get to know one another', and 'have a good time' before they take on the responsibilities of children and childcare (Daniels and Weingarten, 1982; Woollett, Dosanjh-Matwala and Hadlow, 1991). However, there are also pressures not to delay 'too long' the birth of a first child. Insofar as children are seen as an essential step in the establishment or the natural progression of a relationship, a long delay may be seen as a lack of commitment by one or both partners or an unwillingness to 'settle down' and take on the responsibilities of adult life. Women's responses to questions about the timing or spacing of children also indicate that some women want to have children soon after marriage/establishment of a relationship because of their concerns about getting 'too old' to have children or about their fertility. Because of fears about possible effects of contraception on fertility, some women prefer not to use contraception even if it means having children very quickly after entering a relationship (Woollett, Dosanjh-Matwala and Hadlow, 1991).

For some women the timing of a first pregnancy is a result of a conscious decision to have a child and involves deciding to cease using contraception with the aim of becoming pregnant, often referred to as 'trying for a baby'. Other women decide less deliberately that they do not mind whether or not they become pregnant at this point. This may indicate an ambivalence or uncertainty about becoming a mother or when to become a mother, or a more general sense of not being able to control this aspect of their lives (Christopher, 1991; Lees, 1993). Other pregnancies are unplanned and unwanted: about one-third of British pregnancies are unintended and even when it is available, contraception is not necessarily practised or practised effectively (Boyle, 1991; Christopher, 1991). Young and/or single women may not use contraception effectively because of concerns about their health or because they fear being labelled as 'slags' if they try to ensure that they or their partners use contraception (Lees, 1993).

Age at which to have children

Most women in the developed world have their first babies in their twenties or early thirties, at a somewhat later age than was the case in the past. Only about 8% of babies in the UK are born to women under the age of 20, fewer than at any time this century. In contrast the numbers of women in the developed world having a first baby after the age of 30 are increasing (Berryman, 1991; Phoenix, 1991a). Alongside these changes are strongly articulated views about the appropriate age at which to have a first baby. It is often argued that it is best for the baby and for the mother if women have their first babies in their twenties or early thirties and that childbearing is completed before the age of forty (Phoenix and Woollett, 1991).

Women having children before the age of 20 are seen therefore as 'too young' to have children, although there is little evidence to suggest that their age is directly related to any of the problems usually assumed to be associated with young motherhood (Phoenix, 1991b). In the UK, insofar as age is problematic, it is because younger women are more likely to be having first babies (whose deliveries tend to be more problematic than those of later babies), to be single and less financially secure (Phoenix, 1991b).

Even though the number of British women having babies over the age of 35 is increasing, they represent only about 10% of mothers. Women having babies at this age are viewed as 'problematic' because their pregnancies are considered as potentially more complex and the chances of giving birth to a baby with Down's syndrome increases with age. There is, however, little evidence of psychological problems amongst older mothers and their children (Berryman, 1991). The decision to postpone motherhood is often a conscious choice. Women may delay parenthood because they are committed to other activities or are not in relationships in which they feel able/ready to have a child at a younger age. Women (and men) who delay having children tend to be more highly educated, to have experienced a broken marriage and to have married later (Kiernan, 1989). Late motherhood may also result from women being unable to become mothers at an earlier age because of problems in conceiving or carrying a pregnancy to term (Berryman, 1991).

Decisions about family size

Families are often perceived as consisting of parents and two or more children, with families being smaller in European countries such as Italy and Germany and larger in African countries. Two opposing sets of ideas seem to be at work in decisions about family size. Larger families are often considered to create a better environment for child rearing, providing children with opportunities for growing up alongside brothers and sisters. Only-children are often viewed as lonely, missing out on the bustle, excitement and stimulation of family life, selfish and not well adjusted because they do not have to learn to share. There is no evidence to support this negative view of only-children (Laybourn, 1990), but it maintains a powerful influence on people's reproductive decision-making.

On the other hand, there are sometimes strong prescriptions against families which are 'too large', although what is meant by 'large' varies from country to country and often for different religious, ethnic and social class groupings. Negative ideas about large families are based on concerns about the costs of looking after children or being able to provide good marriage settlements. Because children have to share their parents' attention, large families are some-times seen as less stimulating and as providing less impetus for children's development. Accounts of children's psychological development, based on research in developed countries, stress the value of close mother–child relations and maternal sensitivity, but there is little evidence to suggest that large families per se offer a less stimulating environment for children (Woollett, Dosanjh-Matwala and Hadlow, 1991). Despite concerns about the 'problematic' nature of large families, based on their religion (e.g. Catholic), ethnicity (Afro-Caribbean) or both (Asian Muslim), the main problems for large families in the UK are financial (Butler and Golding, 1986; Phoenix, 1990).

Children's gender

Another reason why only children are viewed negatively is because 'proper' families are seen as having a mix of boys and girls (Busfield, 1974). Families with only-children are 'deviant' in respect of their size but also because they include children of only one gender. Parents have strong desires for a mix of boys and girls: there is some evidence to suggest that parents with two boys or two girls are more likely to have a third child than parents with one boy and one girl (Williamson, 1976; Woollett, Dosanjh-Matwala and Hadlow, 1991). These preferences about a mix of boys and girls are often linked with ideas about gender-related activities. Fathers explain their desires for boys in terms of the companionship they expect through engagement in joint activities with boys (Owens, 1982). And mothers' desires for a girl are explained in similar terms, 'someone to do things with', 'similar interests' and hence 'companionship' (McGuire, 1991; Newson and Newson, 1968; Woollett and Phoenix, 1996). Because of this preference about a gender mix, parents are more concerned about the gender of a second than a first child (Woollett, Dosanjh-Matwala and Hadlow, 1991).

Spacing of children

There are strong ideological/cultural beliefs about the spacing of a second and subsequent children (Daniels and Weingarten, 1982; Woollett and Phoenix, 1991; Busfield, 1974). As has already been suggested, the timing of a first birth is often related to a couple's decision to start a family or to ideas about the progress of their relationship. In contrast, the timing of the birth of a second (and subsequent) child is often related to the work of caring for two or more young children. A short gap between children means hard work for mothers but if a second birth is delayed, mothers sometimes say they find it difficult to readjust to the work of caring for a small baby after a break. Mothers may also discuss what they consider to be the benefits of spacing births for children's development: a small age gap between children is linked to the companionship between children and a wider gap to providing each child with sufficient attention (Woollett, Dosanjh-Matwala and Hadlow, 1991). But mothers' ideas are also related to factors such as their age, with older mothers considering that they are less able to delay the birth of a second child than younger mothers. Women's reproductive decisions also relate to whether or not they consider their family to be complete: women who want another child at some stage are less concerned about the efficiency of a contraceptive method than women who consider their families are complete (Thomas, 1985).

How decisions are made

As has been indicated, people make a range of reproductive decisions. These decisions are often complex and sometimes contradictory and not easily explained in 'rational' terms. Their explanations may reflect the extent to which their ideas are 'normative' and shared by the communities in which they live and the extent to which their circumstances mean that they need to explain and give accounts of their decisions. When their choices and preferences are similar to those currently seen as 'normal' and 'natural', women and men have little need to articulate their reasons and hence may have little experience in doing so. When this is the case, their ability to give clear accounts of their reproductive decisions may be an indication of people's linguistic skills or their experience of articulating their ideas and their feelings generally rather than the rationality of their reproductive decision-making.

People are often asked to consider their reproductive decisions using dichotomous categories: pregnancies are 'planned *or* unplanned', 'wanted *or* unwanted'. In contrast research which allows people to answer such questions more fully makes it clear that either/or categories are inappropriate because they do not respect the complexity and ambivalence of people's decisions. The picture is further complicated because people's accounts are usually given after the event and hence represent post hoc rationalizations or attempts to impose meaning upon events rather than indicating the ideas and choices which were perhaps salient when people made their decisions (Porter, 1991; Sheeran, White and Phillips, 1991).

The complexity of people's decision-making and the inappropriateness of these dichotomous ways of conceptualizing decisions has been demonstrated in a number of studies. Phoenix (1991b), for example, found some consistency between the extent to which single young women felt it was important not to get pregnant, their use of contraception, and their feelings when they discovered they were pregnant. But often their replies to questions about these aspects of their decision-making were not easily categorized. Similar problems were encountered in Wolkind and Zajicek's (1981) study of single and married women expecting their first babies. While those women who said their pregnancies were planned were somewhat more likely to report positive feelings, this was by no means always the case: women's feelings sometimes changed over time, often related to changes in their circumstances and/or the severity of their pregnancy symptoms.

As this chapter has indicated, more is known about the reproductive decisions of women than men. This reflects the greater impact on women's lives of the technologies available to control fertility and the changes which motherhood brings to women's lives and identities. Lewis (1982) reported that men felt that it was their wives/partners who made the decision to become pregnant and that men had a more peripheral role, but women's accounts do suggest that they are aware and take note of men's ideas and preferences (Woollett and Phoenix, 1991). Even though this is an important aspect of reproductive decision-making, there is little research which helps us to understand how men and women negotiate their reproductive decisions and their choice of methods of contraception/fertility control (Porter, 1991).

Reproductive decision-making is largely a personal concern for the women (and where applicable, the men) involved but these private decisions are made within the context of a framework of ideas about the value of children, family size and composition and the context in which children should be conceived and brought up (New and David, 1985; Phoenix and Woollett, 1991). These ideologies around children, families and parenthood influence public policy and the provision of services which facilitate or make it difficult for people to translate their choices and preferences into practice. For example, contraception services are targeted according to public definitions of needs/problems and hence at groups (such as Asian families in the UK) where 'large' families are considered more prevalent rather than at women under the age of 16 where it is feared that the provision of contraception may legitimize 'under age' (and hence 'problematic') sexual activity (Phoenix, 1990). Similarly, it is often argued that adoption and infertility services should be available only to those who are deemed suitable as parents (that is married couples or those in stable heterosexual relations) rather than according to the needs and preferences of individual men and women (Phoenix and Woollett, 1991).

Applications

1. There is a need to understand how women and men make their reproductive decisions. This understanding should not be influenced by findings obtained from non-normative groups such as infertile men and women, when the decisions and choices of women and men in different circumstances are being addressed.

2. Increased recognition needs to be given to the variability, complexity and inconsistencies apparent in reproductive decision-making.

3. There should be an awareness that ideas about children, families and the circumstances in which children 'should' be brought up are changing and may not equate with pre-existing ideas expressed in the literature or by practitioners.

Further reading

Michaels, G. Y. (1988). Motivational factors in the decision and timing of pregnancy. In *Transition to parenthood: theory and research* (G. Y. Michaels and W. A. Goldberg, eds). Cambridge: Cambridge University Press.

Phoenix, A., Woollett, A. and Lloyd, E. (eds) (1991). *Motherhood: meanings, practices and ideologies*. London: Sage.

Special issue of *Journal of Reproductive and Infant Psychology*, Volume 9, issue 4, 1991 'Family Planning and Reproductive Decisions' edited by A. Walker and E. McNeil.

References

Antonis, B. (1981). Motherhood and mothering. In *Women in Society* (Cambridge Women's Studies Group, ed) London: Virago.

Berryman, J. C. (1991). Perspectives on later motherhood. In *Motherhood: meanings, practices and ideologies* (A. Phoenix, A. Woollett and E. Lloyd, eds). London: Sage.

Boulton, G. M. (1983). *On being a mother: a study of women with preschool children*. London: Tavistock.

Boyle, M. (1991). Decision making for contraception and abortion. In *Psychology and Health* (M. Pitts and K. Phillips, eds). London: Routledge.

Busfield, J. (1974). Ideologies and reproduction. In *The integration of the child into a social world* (M. Richards, ed.). Cambridge: Cambridge University Press.

Butler, N. R. and Golding, J. (eds) (1986). *From birth to five: a study of the health and behaviour of Britain's five year olds*. Oxford: Pergamon.

Calvert, B. and Stanton, W. R. (1992). Perspectives of parenthood: similarities and differences between 15-year-old girls and boys. *Adolescence*, **27**, 106, 315–28.

Campbell, E. (1985). *The childless marriage: an exploratory study of couples who do not want children*. London: Tavistock.

Christopher, E. (1991). Family planning and reproductive decisions. *Journal of Reproductive and Infant Psychology*, **9**, 217–26.

Croghan, R. (1991). First-time mothers' accounts of inequality in the division of labour. *Feminism and Psychology*, **1**, 221–46.

Daniels, P. and Weingarten, K. (1982). *Sooner or later*. New York: W W Norton.

Fawcett, J. T. (1988). The value of children and the transition to parenthood. *Marriage and Family Review*, **12**, 12–34.

Franklin, S. (1989). Deconstructing 'desperateness': the social construction of infertility in popular representations of new reproductive technologies. In *The New Reproductive technologies* (M. McNeil, I. Varcoe and S. Yearley, eds). London: Macmillan.

Greenberger, E. and Goldberg, W. A. (1989). Work, parenting and the socialization of children. *Developmental Psychology*, **25**, 22–35.

Hubert, J. (1974). Belief and reality: social factors in pregnancy and childbirth. In *Integration of the child into a social world* (M. Richards, ed.) London: Cambridge University Press.

Kiernan, K. (1989). Who remains childless? *Journal of Biosocial Science*, **21**, 387–98.

Laybourn, A. (1990). Only children in Britain: popular stereotypes and research evidence. *Children and Society*, **4**, 386–400.

Lees, S. (1993). *Sugar and spice: sexuality and adolescent girls*. Harmondsworth: Penguin.

Lewis, C. (1982). 'A feeling you can't scratch'?: The effect of pregnancy and birth on married men. In *Fathers: psychological perspectives* (N. Beail and J. McGuire, eds). London: Junction Books.

Lewis, S. (1991). Motherhood and employment: the impact of social and organisational values. In *Motherhood: meanings, practices and ideologies* (A. Phoenix, A. Woollett and E. Lloyd, eds). London: Sage.

Llewelyn, S. and Osborne, K. (1990). *Women's lives*. London: Routledge.

Mason, M.-C. (1993). *Male infertility: men talking*. London: Routledge.

McGuire, J. (1991). Sons and daughters. In *Motherhood: meanings, practices and ideologies* (A. Phoenix, A. Woollett and E. Lloyd, eds). London: Sage.

Michaels, G. Y. (1988). Motivational factors in the decision and timing of pregnancy. In *Transition to parenthood: theory and research* (G. Y. Michaels and W. A. Goldberg, eds). Cambridge: Cambridge University Press.

New, C. and David, M. (1985). *For the children's sake: making childcare more than women's business*. Harmondsworth: Penguin.

Newson, J. and Newson, E. (1968). *Four Years Old in an urban community*. Harmondsworth: Penguin.

Oakley, A. (1981). *Becoming a mother: from here to maternity*. Harmondsworth: Penguin.

Owens, D. (1982). The desire to father: reproductive ideologies and involuntarily childless men. In *The Father Figure* (L. McKee and M. O'Brien, eds). London: Tavistock.

Payne, J. (1978). Talking about children: an examination of accounts about reproduction and family life. *Journal of Biosocial Science*, **10**, 367–74.

Pfeffer, N. and Woollett, A. (1983). *The Experience of Infertility*. London: Virago.

Phoenix, A. (1990). Black women and the maternity services. In *The politics of maternity of care: services for childbearing women in twentieth-century Britain* (J. Garcia, M. P. M. Richards and R. Kilpatrick, eds). Oxford: Clarendon Press.

Phoenix, A. (1991a). Mothers under twenty: outsider and insider views. In *Motherhood: meanings, practices and ideologies* (A. Phoenix, A. Woollett and E. Lloyd, eds). London: Sage.

Phoenix, A. (1991b). *Young mothers?* Cambridge: Polity.

Phoenix, A. and Woollett, A. (1991). Motherhood: Social Construction, Politics and Psychology. In *Motherhood: meanings, practices and ideologies* (A. Phoenix, A. Woollett and E. Lloyd, eds). London: Sage.

Phoenix, A., Woollett, A. and Lloyd, E. (eds) (1991) *Motherhood: meanings, practices and ideologies*. London: Sage.

Porter, M. (1991). Contraceptive choices: an exploratory study of how they are made. *Journal of Reproductive and Infant Psychology*, **9**, 227–36.

Sheeran, P., White, D. and Phillips, K. (1991). Premarital contraceptive use: a review of the psychological literature. *Journal of Reproductive and Infant Psychology*, **9**, 253–69.

Thomas, H. (1985). The medical construction of the contraceptive career. In *The sexual politics of reproduction* (H. Homans, ed). Aldershot: Gower.

Veevers, J. E. (1980). *Childless by choice*. Toronto: Butterworths.

Westwood, S. and Bhachu, P. (eds) (1988). *Enterprising Women: Ethnicity, economy and gender relations*. London: Routledge.

Williamson, N. (1976). *Sons or daughters? A cross-cultural study of parental preferences*. London: Sage.

Wolkind, S. and Zajicek, E. (1981). *Pregnancy: a psychological and social study*. London: Academic Press.

Woollett, A. (1991). Having children: accounts of childless women and women with reproductive problems. In *Motherhood: meanings, practices and ideologies* (A. Phoenix, A. Woollett and E. Lloyd, eds). London: Sage.

Woollett, A. (1992). Young people's ideas about families: a context for reproductive decision making. Annual Conference of the Society for Reproductive and Infant Psychology, University of Strathclyde, September.

Woollett, A., Dosanjh-Matwala, N. and Hadlow, J. (1991). Reproductive decision making: Asian women's ideas about family size, and the gender and spacing of children. *Journal of Reproductive and Infant Psychology*, **9**, 237–52.

Woollett, A. and Phoenix, A. (1991) Psychological views of mothering. In *Motherhood: meanings, practices and ideologies* (A. Phoenix, A. Woollett and E. Lloyd, eds). London: Sage.

Woollett, A. and Phoenix, A. (1996). Motherhood as pedagogy: developmental psychology and the accounts of mothers of young children. In *Feminisms and the pedagogies of everyday life* (C. Luke, ed). New York: State University of New York.

2

Infertility

Josephine Emery

> In Chapter 1, the factors underlying the decision to reproduce were discussed. However, not every couple who decides to 'try for a baby' will conceive. As Jo Emery reports in this chapter, about 15% of couples will experience some problems with their fertility. Psychological factors have been implicated as one possible cause of infertility, and it is increasingly recognized that infertility and its diagnosis and treatment can result in psychological distress. The author discusses the circularity of this cause-and-effect cycle and the complexity of the inter-relationship between psychological and biological factors.
>
> The consideration of infertility in Chapter 2 leads into the following chapter which looks at the impact that the new reproductive technologies have in resolving this problem.

Introduction

The diagnosis of infertility is typically a lengthy and rather unpleasant process, involving intimate examination, personal enquiry and, frequently, invasive procedures. The causes of infertility established by the diagnostic process include ovulatory disorder (30%), sperm defects and disorders (each about 25%) and tubal/pelvic disorder usually resulting from infection (20%). Less frequent causes include endometriosis, cervical mucus defects or disorders and coital impairment (Hull, 1992). Thus most cases of infertility may be attributed to a specific organic cause with a recognized pathology (termed organic infertility). However around 25% of infertility is unexplained. Infertility may also be primary, for example in women when menstruation has never occurred or in men where there is azoospermia, or secondary when potential reproductive functioning has been established but for some reason ceases.

While debate surrounds the epidemiology of infertility, recently Templeton, Fraser and Thompson (1991) have suggested an overall infertility rate of 15%. Rates of infertility are not, however, stable. They are affected by the availability of effective contraception which allows couples to space their families and in many cases now to postpone parenthood past the age of peak reproductive capacity. This tends to increase overall rates of infertility. However, conversely it also has the effect of increasing fertility in women in their thirties and forties (Botting, 1992). Another factor which is currently acting to increase infertility levels is the considerable increase in sexually transmitted disease which leads to pelvic infection (Templeton, 1992).

Recent advances in the treatment of infertility, and media interest in the new reproductive technologies, discussed in Chapter 3, have served to increase public awareness of infertility. In this chapter the psychological impact of infertility will be examined since a precise understanding of the effects of infertility, infertility investigation and treatment is imperative if appropriate cost-effective services are to be provided, not just in terms of medical treatment but also with regard to psychological well-being which may influence effective treatment outcome. With this objective in mind, the current literature will be reviewed focusing on the areas of emotional, sexual and marital functioning. The influence that stress may have on infertility will be debated since the possibility arises that the effects of stress may act to reduce fertility, and the coping and adjustment of infertile couples will be discussed in this context.

Emotional aspects of infertility

In contrast to the changing epidemiology of infertility and the improvements in treatment regimens, there has been little change in social attitudes towards those who are unable to reproduce. As Chapter 1 has discussed, society contrives to impose two major norms with regard to fertility: the expectation that all couples should reproduce at some stage within their partnership and that such couples should want to produce offspring (Rosenfeld and Mitchell, 1979; Veevers, 1980). Childlessness, whether voluntary or not is viewed as a form of deviant behaviour (Miall, 1985). Consequently infertile couples face enormous pressure from family, friends and society at large to conform to the expectations of procreation (Muller, 1985).

Furthermore, infertility involves a traumatic event initiated by the lack of a viable pregnancy; intensified by the confirmation of a diagnosis and requiring a major adjustment in life. Infertile couples additionally experience a chronic ongoing series of pressures and inconveniences largely attributable to the plethora of medical procedures to which they are exposed (Kraft, Palombo and Mitchell, 1980; Mahlstedt, 1985). Consequently, there appears to be little doubt among clinicians and others that infertility incorporates the experience of stress at some level. If the construct of stress is viewed as having two main components, stressors which are the external physical stimuli, and the stress response which is manifested in the reactive patterns consisting of physiological, cognitive and behavioural components (Feuerstein, Labbe and Kuczmierczyk, 1986), then in some way it will affect the infertile couple's life. Such reactions may include significantly raised levels of anxiety or depression. There may also be a variety of behavioural and personality manifestations, varying along a continuum from mild to severe and from normal to maladjusted.

Much of the available research literature purports to depict the range of emotional reactions to infertility. However this literature is dominated by retrospective and often anecdotal accounts of couples' reactions, and its findings may also be influenced by couples' attempts to portray their psychological functioning in a positive light because they fear that otherwise they may be excluded from treatment. There is a clear need for well-designed prospective studies which can accurately reflect any changes which occur in psychological functioning as investigation and treatment progress.

Many infertile women describe the initial investigations and treatment as being the most upsetting experience of their lives (Freeman, Boxer, Rickets et al., 1985). Indeed 63% rated infertility as more stressful than divorce, where both had been experienced (Mahlstedt, Macduff and Bernstein, 1987). Denial of a life option always taken for granted can stir a powerful anger. A personal sense of justice is violated, leading to feelings of frustration and in some cases to rage and acting-out behaviour (Bresnick and Taymor, 1979; Kraft, Palombo and Mitchell,

1980; Mahlstedt, 1985; Moos and Schaefer, 1986). However, other couples behave differently, avoiding any discussion of infertility even between themselves and demonstrating resigned acceptance (Callan, 1988; Callan and Hennessy, 1988b). Some though not all couples have been found to express jealousy of couples with children and to radically restructure their lives in order to avoid any contact with pregnancy, babies or children (Mahlstedt, 1985; Menning, 1980). Social isolation from friends and family can occur because they demonstrate a lack of insight into the emotional aspects of infertility and make insensitive remarks, such as expressing surprise that a child has not been produced. This can lead to the infertile couple losing their sense of control over their lives and hesitating to confide in family and friends which in turn tends to reduce sources of support (Bierkens, 1973; Lalos, Lalos, Jacobsonn and Schultz, 1985; Platt, Fischer and Silver, 1973). This self-imposed isolation may also generate feelings of being 'defective' with a consequent lowering of self-esteem and coping ability (Mahlstedt, 1985; Mazor, 1984). In such circumstances there is a clear need for professional supportive counselling, a need recognized by infertile couples themselves (Lalos, Lalos, Jacobsonn and Schultz, 1985), since social support is positively related to recovery from stressful life events in general and, in infertility, is associated with the continuation of treatment (Callan and Hennessy, 1989).

Infertility also involves many kinds of loss, each of which can contribute to the development of anxiety or depression (Mahlstedt, 1985). Lack of biological parenthood can lead to a grief reaction that is unique to the extent that it is a loss concerned with what might have been rather than with what was; the infertile couple having lost the potential to become parents (Daniels, Gumby, Legge et al., 1984). Grieving can be helpful in allowing the couple to adapt emotionally to the impact of infertility (Callan, 1988). However, it can be hindered by the maintenance of hope that pregnancy may occur, and the private nature of infertility and the social isolation of infertile couples can result in unrecognized and unresolved grieving which is difficult to identify clinically and even more problematic to resolve (Mahlstedt, 1985).

The findings reviewed so far might be taken to suggest that infertility invariably leads to negative emotional reactions and poor psychological well-being. It is therefore important to recognize that in studies where infertile and fertile subject groups are compared there is often little evidence of significant differences, except when there is a long history of infertility and treatment (e.g. Slade, 1981). Furthermore, research involving infertile couples who are engaged in IVF treatment consistently shows these couples to be well adjusted (e.g. Freeman, Boxer, Rickels et al., 1985; see Chapter 3).

Gender differences have been found in many studies of emotional reaction to infertility. For example Lalos, Lalos, Jacobsonn and Schultz (1985) found that infertile women were more likely to admit to a range of symptoms including grief, depression, guilt, feelings of inferiority and isolation, than their partners. Raval, Slade, Buck and Lieberman (1987) found infertile women more likely to experience anxiety and depression at levels above population norms in comparison to their partners, and similar results were demonstrated in studies by Andrews, Abbey and Halman (1992). A relatively large-scale study which compared 335 infertile women and 38 fertile controls on standardized measures of depression again found twice the levels of depressive symptoms in the infertile group (Domar, Broome, Zuttermeister et al., 1992). Thus research which compares female infertile subjects with fertile controls seems more likely to detect significant differences between the populations. Domar, Broome, Zuttermeister et al. (1992) however found that levels of anxiety in their female infertile group could be predicted by low frequency of sexual intercourse, a finding which is comparable to that of Kedem, Mikulinger and Nathanson (1990) in a study concerned with male infertility, where increased anxiety and feelings of hopelessness were related to sexual inadequacy. Thus gender differences are not always apparent and where found may be related to more generalized aspects of gender and health, for example in depression, rather than in areas specific to infertility.

Within the specific context of infertility, studies have sought to examine whether differences in psychological measures are related to diagnostic category. If found, such differences might suggest that some forms of infertility, most notably those categorized as 'non-organic' or 'unexplained', were a consequence of maladaptive psychological functioning rather than a cause (Paulson, Haarmann, Salerno and Asmar, 1988). Studies reviewed by Edelmann and Connolly (1986) found no differences in personality measures between organic and non-organic infertility groups but did find that heightened anxiety was more likely in subjects with a diagnosis of 'unexplained' infertility. These findings taken together with the results of studies which have found no relationship between emotional maladjustment and infertility, or between anxiety levels and the subsequent resolution of infertility, cast doubt on the historical view that psychological factors are causal in infertility (Edelmann, Connolly, Cooke and Robson, 1991; Paulson, Haarmann, Salerno and Asmar, 1988).

However, it remains possible that any stress and distress which develops as a consequence of infertility may exacerbate or interact with causal organic factors. A number of researchers have noted the effects of stressful stimuli on female hormone secretions. For instance, stress-induced hypersecretion of prolactin can affect follicular maturation and the subsequent luteal phase which leads to ovulation. By suppressing the positive feedback of oestrogens that are responsible for the lutenizing hormone surge, the ovum may not be released from the follicle since the latter fails to mature. This psychobiological mechanism is referred to as stress-induced hyperprolactinaemia. Some support for the hypothesized effects of this mechanism in unexplained infertility in women has been provided by Edelmann and Golombok (1989). However, although evidence is available that infertility is associated with high psychological stress, for example from a two-year prospective study of 71 couples (Moller and Fallstrom, 1991); and that infertile women with luteal phase insufficiency suffer from high anxiety and employ less effective strategies in coping with stress and anxiety (Pesch, Weyer and Taubert, 1989), conclusive evidence of a direct link between infertility, stress, coping and hyperprolactinaemia cannot be demonstrated until psychological and endocrinological research are carried out in tandem.

Issues of timing are also crucial. An interesting study by Berg and Wilson (1991) appraised psychological, marital and sexual adjustment in a cross-sectional study of 104 couples with a diagnosis of primary infertility who were at one, two and three plus years into treatment. Reviewing other studies, the authors suggested that treatment for infertility may produce both short- and long-term symptoms of psychological and relationship strain. This stage model would predict an acute phase concerned with the stress of diagnosis and early treatment which rapidly subsides, followed by a chronic phase where repeated unsuccessful treatment regimens gradually erode personal and relationship coping resources. Measures used to test this hypothesis included the SCL-90-R (Derogatis, 1983), the Marital Adjustment Test (MAT) and a questionnaire designed to cover relationship and sexual issues. The SCL-90-R results indicated that on measures of depression, hostility, anxiety, phobic anxiety, interpersonal relations, psychoticism, obsession-compulsion, paranoid ideation and somatosization, there was a consistent pattern of increased scores at year one, reduced scores at year two and that the highest scores were recorded at and beyond year three. Relationship scores on the MAT were within the normal range, but with a downward trend so that at the third time point, borderline adjustment scores and reduced marital satisfaction scores were recorded. There was overall sexual satisfaction but a strong linear trend emerged with significantly lower scores at three years plus. Again fluctuations were apparent in both male and female sexual functioning with higher scores two years into treatment and lower scores, for example in ejaculatory control and female orgasm, at year three and beyond. This pattern of fluctuating psychological functioning at the different time points into infertility treatment is consistent with the author's model of infertility strain with an acute stress reaction at diagnosis and initial treatment which diminishes over time, overlaid by a chronic strain response which intensifies as treatment continues. Unfortunately, this study did not employ a control group to assess the effects of time on psychological, marital and sexual functioning in fertile couples. Other longitudinal studies have found evidence of fluctuations in psychological well-being with anxiety being found to increase from before, to after, infertility investigation (Takefman, Brender, Boivin and Tulandi, 1990) and a reduction in active coping and a decrease in sexual activities being found in a prospective study lasting 28 months (Strauss, Appelt, Bohnet and Ulrich, 1992). The results of this latter study showed that infertile women who were assessed as psychologically impaired before treatment was begun, were less likely to become pregnant as a result of treatment. Thus the timing of assessments not only affects the scores obtained on outcome measures of psychological functioning but also may have predictive value for treatment success.

Marital and sexual issues

Estrangement within the marital relationship may occur because the diagnosis of infertility places a severe strain on communication and understanding between the couple. This is especially likely to occur when one partner is identified as the primary cause of the infertility. This partner may experience guilt, and fear of being rejected or abandoned. Even though his or her spouse may appear to be supportive, suppressed feelings of anger and resentment are not uncommon (Mazor, 1984). Greater marital difficulties have also been reported by both men and women when the cause of the infertility can be attributed to the man (Connolly and Edelmann, 1987). However, once again longitudinal studies paint a somewhat different picture with Daniluk (1988) failing to find any evidence of a change in the quality of the relationship in 43 subjects with a diagnosis of primary infertility. Indeed some cases of infertility may serve to cement a relationship. Raval, Slade, Buck and Lieberman (1987) reported a reduction in marital problems experienced by couples after attending an infertility clinic perhaps because some action had been taken to deal with on-going infertility.

Link and Darling (1986) in a survey of 43 couples undergoing infertility investigation, found that 84% of the female subjects and 88% of the males appeared to be experiencing sexual difficulties, as assessed by the Index of Sexual Satisfaction (Hudson and Glisson, 1982). Looking at 71 couples over a two-year period from the time of their first consultation with a doctor regarding their infertility, Moller and Fallstrom (1991) found that although most coped with the stress on their relationship, if a pregnancy had not been established by the time of the final follow up, 25% of the sample felt that their relationship had been impaired to a degree that included sexual problems. Similarly, out of 47 couples studied by Raval, Slade, Buck and Lieberman (1987), two-thirds of the women reported sexual difficulties after the recognition of the infertility, although their partners reported fewer sexual problems (this may be because women have a greater psychological investment in reproduction compared with men (Greenglass, 1982)).

It has also been suggested that a diagnosis of unexplained infertility has particular implications for poor sexual adjustment (Daniluk, 1988). Takefman, Brender, Boivin and Tulandi (1990) found that sexual difficulties with low intercourse frequency, together with poor marital adjustment and higher psychological distress, may be predictors of poorer adjustment to infertility.

Furthermore, as discussed above, there is evidence that the sexual relationship may deteriorate, particularly as medical interventions progress (Berg and Wilson, 1991; McGrade and Tolor, 1981). Problems such as impotence can appear mid-cycle when the chances of conceiving are highest and couples need to feel at their most responsive (Drake and Grunert, 1979). Concerns about sexual inadequacy may develop even though couples recognize that fertility and sexuality are separate issues (Mazor, 1984). Sexual dysfunction may be thought to be the cause of infertility and feelings of sexual unattractiveness can ensue (Rosenfeld and Mitchell, 1979) leading to concerns about actual performance technique (Seibel and Taymor, 1982). There is also an indication that in an attempt to gain verification of their potency and desirability, extra-relationship flirtations may occur and affairs can follow (Kraft, Palombo and Mitchell, 1980). Accordingly, counselling needs have been discussed by Van Zyl (1987) who found that out of 514 couples, 42% had psychosexual problems that were causing emotional distress. He suggested that sex education as well as counselling could be beneficial.

Coping and infertility

Throughout the 1970s there was a growing conviction that coping with stress affected psychological, physical and social well-being (see Antonovsky, 1979, for a review). The conceptualization of coping that emerged from this body of research concentrated on the cognitive-phenomenological theory of psychological stress developed by Folkman and Lazarus (Folkman, 1984). Within this theory, the individual and the environment are seen as being in a relationship of on-going reciprocal action, each affecting the other in turn, where appraisal and coping appear to mediate their interaction. Appraisal is the cognitive process through which an event is evaluated with respect to the relative importance of the situation, and is referred to as primary appraisal. The diversity of coping resource options that are available is known as secondary appraisal. The level of stress experienced depends on the evaluation of the importance of the event and the range of coping options. Coping may, therefore, be defined as 'the cognitive and behavioural efforts made to master, tolerate or reduce external and/or internal demands and conflicts amongst them' (Folkman and Lazarus, 1980). The management or alteration of the person–environment relationship that is the source of stress may be regarded as problem-focused coping. The regulation of stressful emotions is referred to as emotion-focused coping. Folkman and Lazarus (1980) showed that both forms of coping are used in most stressful encounters and that the relative proportions of each vary according to the appraisal of the situation.

Apart from these relational aspects of the cognitive theory of stress and coping, a process-oriented theory has also been developed (Folkman, 1984). This has two implications: that an individual is in a dynamic relationship with the environment and, that this relationship is bi-directional. As the relationship orientation of coping intimates that personal control must be viewed in the context of a particular person–environment interaction, then the idea of process indicates that appraisals of personal control are likely to change throughout a stressful encounter as a result of changes in the person–environment relationship (Folkman, 1984). Thus perceptions of control need to be examined in the context of each specific stressful encounter.

Within the person–environment model of coping (Folkman, 1984), infertility can be interpreted as a threat to personal well-being which can be viewed as stressful. As many studies have shown, infertility is usually accompanied by a sense of personal loss (e.g. Pfeffer and Woollett, 1983) which may be regarded as a primary appraisal. However, it could also be appraised more positively as a challenge to which the couple can respond. Secondary appraisal arises due to the fact that the stresses associated with infertility require individuals to evaluate their coping options. The length of time involved in investigations and treatment also indicates that these options may need to be reappraised for instance in response to years of unsuccessful treatment. This reappraisal may also involve some re-evaluation of the success of coping strategies (Callan and Hennessey, 1988a).

With regard to control, the cognitive-based model of coping presented here would predict that the infertile couple would employ appraisal together with problem-focused and emotion-focused coping. Appraisal is necessary in order to understand the crisis of infertility and will be affected by the introduction of new information as the couple's knowledge base extends. Problem-focused coping allows confrontation of the problem in an attempt to establish a solution, along with the consideration of alternative strategies to achieve this goal. Emotion-focused coping requires the couple to deal with the emotional impact of a diagnosis of infertility, the inherent demands of treatment and cognitive attempts to accept the infertility per se.

A study of 76 females and 54 males who had been trying to conceive over a one-year period utilized the cognitive model of stress by focusing on cognitive appraisal and adjustment to infertility (Stanton, Tennen, Affleck and Mendola, 1991). Measures of cognitive appraisal, global distress (SCL-90-R) and infertility-specific distress were used. Outcome showed that infertile subjects were more distressed than the normative sample with women reporting greater infertility-specific distress than their husbands. On measures of appraisal, females who were more threatened or less challenged or who perceived themselves as having less control over their infertility problems, were more distressed. Cognitive appraisals were unrelated to distress in males. However, husbands reported less distress when their wives perceived infertility as a greater challenge.

A further study informed by the cognitive coping framework used a sample of 96 females and 72 males, also having attempted conception for one year (Stanton, Tennen, Affleck and Mendola, 1992). Subjects completed the Ways of Coping Questionnaire (Folkman, Lazarus, Dunkel-Schetter, Delongis and Gruen, 1986) and the SCL-90-R (Derogatis, 1983). Analysis supported the view that multiple coping strategies are used in dealing with infertility. Eighty-eight per cent of males and 94% of females used seven out of the eight coping strategies described by the Ways of Coping Questionnaire. Levels of distress indicated that 32% of males and 35% of females had scores one standard deviation above the standardization means for the SCL-90-R. Few male coping scores were related to distress, with only avoidance and distress being significantly associated. Female coping scores, however did significantly predict distress. When their pattern of coping involved accepting responsibility for the infertility, levels of distress were increased, whereas seeking social support tended to reduce distress. Within the couples, wives were less likely than their partners to cope through distancing, self-control and planful problem solving and were more likely than their spouses to use social support and to cope through escape–avoidance. While couples did not differ in terms of global distress, wives who used self-control had partners who scored more highly for distress. Interestingly the authors concluded that an increase in any coping strategy appeared to be related to greater distress, although further research appears necessary to clarify this point since the definitions of coping utilized in the Ways of Coping Questionnaire may reflect negative responses to stress rather than positive coping efforts.

A more positive view of coping was taken by Callan and Hennessey (1989) who reviewed a range of possible coping strategies that couples might have employed in coping with infertility, thus attempting to utilize the cognitive model of coping in a practical context. A multivariate array of strategies emerged, including seeking information or social support; using denial and delay in seeking treatment to provide temporary relief; breaking the overwhelming impact of the diagnosis into manageable steps; positive thinking; calm acceptance with some degree of detachment; comparison with real or imaginary others which would allow infertility to be perceived as more treatable; taking action particularly by joining an IVF programme which could have the additional benefit of reducing isolation; and looking at life alternatives to having children.

Conclusion

It does seem that infertile couples experience emotional difficulties which may be precipitated or maintained by the infertility, its investigations and subsequent treatment regimens. Females appear to report a greater number of emotional difficulties than their male counterparts which may embrace anxiety, depression, stress, loss of control, anger, and loss of self-esteem. However, many infertility studies have failed to identify or report specific diagnoses for their samples, length of time since investigations or treatment had commenced and many other factors that might have become intervening variables within the research design. Consequently, it has been problematic to pinpoint cause or effect, and any interpretations of the data must be viewed cautiously, especially as many of the studies looking at infertile couples have failed to utilize reliable standardized measures.

Infertility does not appear to have a major impact on the relationship between couples, and there have been reports of infertility bringing a couple closer together with improved levels of communication. Suggestions have been made that couples are reluctant to divulge any negative effects on their psychosocial state for fear of being excluded from treatment options. Equally importantly, however, it has been noted that a strong relationship is necessary to cope with the demands of infertility, investigations and treatment, and this is especially true for assisted conception (see Chapter 3). In the small subgroup that could be recognized as having relationship problems, it was not clear whether these had arisen as a result of infertility treatment or whether they had been pre-existing.

There are some discrepancies in the literature with regard to sexual functioning, although in general sexual relationships do not appear to be grossly dysfunctional. Again, it is obscure whether problems, where they exist, pre-empted infertility or whether dysfunction results from lack of fertility, and/or the treatment process.

Any event, positive or negative, requires individuals to develop ways of coping. As has become evident from discussion of the coping process, people cope in complex ways that evolve as an event progresses. Studies looking directly at coping mechanisms in infertile individuals are few. What has emerged however, is that there is a need for prospective work that may clarify changes in coping strategies that occur over time. My own recently completed prospective study investigating the psychological aspects of up to three cycles of IVF treatment, indicated that coping with the onerous burden of treatment appears to involve multiple strategies.

Some stability of emotion-focused coping was identified together with fluctuations in problem-focused coping which peaked prior to treatment and were highest before a final IVF attempt. More importantly, those who experienced greatest difficulties in coping appeared to be those who entered the IVF programme with pre-existing psychological distress.

In seeking to understand the psychological impact of infertility from an aetiological point of view, it is probably necessary to postulate explanations involving both cause and effect. It could be argued that a long history of infertility may logically lead to psychological distress. Indeed, in a recent commentary, Paulson and Sauer (1991) noted that cancer and infertility treatments are comparable as both have a definable endpoint: cure and a live birth, respectively. With this in mind, Domar, Zuttermeister and Friedman (1993) have hypothesized that it is the chronicity of a disorder which affects its levels of distress experienced, rather than the diagnosis per se. The results of their study indicated that psychological symptoms associated with infertility were similar to those found in patients with other serious medical conditions such as cancer. However, further prospective studies gathering data from multiple time points during investigation, diagnosis and treatment are required.

Applications

1. Reading (1991) has suggested that intervention strategies for infertile couples should encourage stress reduction and the enhancement of coping skills. This approach is obviously informed by the cognitive coping model of stress and could incorporate the provision of information and more general sex education recommended by other workers in the field of infertility.

2. The primary aim of those working with infertile couples should be to prevent the development or exacerbation of adverse psychological reactions at all stages of investigation and treatment. Counselling may help in this regard but many couples may not require such input.

Further reading

Stanton, A. L. and Dunkel-Schetter, C. (eds) (1991). *Infertility: Perspectives from Stress and Coping Research.* New York: Plenum press.

Tan, S. L. and Jacobs, H. S. (1991). *Infertility: Your Questions Answered.* New York, McGraw-Hill. (A useful book for infertile couples.)

Templeton, A. A. and Drife, J. O. (eds) (1992). *Infertility.* New York, Springer-Verlag.

References

Andrews, F. M., Abbey, A. and Halman, L. J. (1992). Is fertility-problem stress different? The dynamics of stress in fertile and infertile couples. *Fertility and Sterility*, **57**, 1247–53.

Antonovsky, A. (1979). Health, Stress and Coping. San Francisco: Jossey-Bass.

Berg, B. J. and Wilson, J. F. (1991). Psychological Functioning Across Stages of Treatment for Infertility. *Journal of Behavioural Medicine*, **14** (1) 11–26.

Bierkens, P. B. (1973). Childlessness From the Psychological Point of View. *Bulletin of the Menninger Clinic*, **39**, (2), 177–82.

Botting, B. J. (1992). Reproductive Trends in the UK. In *Infertility* (A. A. Templeton and J. O. Drife, eds). New York, Springer-Verlag

Bresnick, E. and Taymor, M. L. (1979). The role of counselling in infertility. *Fertility and Sterility*, **32**, 154–6.

Callan, V. J. (1988). *Infertility: A Guide for Couples.* Melbourne: Pitman.

Callan, V. J. and Hennessey, J. F. (1988a). Emotional Aspects and Support in In-Vitro Fertilization and Embryo Transfer Programs. *Journal of In-Vitro Fertilization and Embryo Transfer*, **5**, (5), 290–95.

Callan, V. J. and Hennessey, J. F. (1988b). The psychological adjustment of women experiencing infertility. *British Journal of Medical Psychology*, **61**, 137–40.

Callan, V. J. and Hennessey, J. F. (1989). Strategies for coping with infertility. *British Journal of Medical Psychology*, **62**, 343–54.

Connolly, K. J. and Edelmann, R. J. (1987). Distress and marital problems associated with infertility: a preliminary investigation. *Journal of Reproductive and Infant Psychology*, **5**, (1), 49–57.

Daniels, K. R., Gumby, J., Legge, M., Williams, T. and Wynn-Williams, D. B. (1984). Issues and Problems for the Infertile Couple. *New Zealand Medical Journal*, **97**, 185–7.

Daniluk, J. (1988). Infertility: intrapersonal and interpersonal impact. *Fertility and Sterility*, **49**, (6), 982–90.

Derogatis, L. (1983). SCL-90-R: Administration, Scoring and Procedures Manual II for the Revised Version and Other Instruments of the Psychopathology Rating Scale Series, 2nd edn. Towson, MD: Clinical Psychometric Research.

Domar, A. D., Broome, A., Zuttermeister, P. C., Seibel, M. M. and Friedman, R. (1992). The prevalence and predictability of depression in infertile women. *Fertility and Sterility*, **58**, 1158–61.

Domar, A. D., Zuttermeister, P. C.and Friedman, R. (1993). The psychological impact of infertility: a comparison with patients with other medical conditions. *Journal of Psychosomatic Obstetrics and Gynaecology*, **14**, Special Issue, 45–52.

Drake, T. S. and Grunert, G. M. (1979). A cyclic pattern of sexual dysfunction in the infertility investigation. *Fertility and Sterility*, **32**, 542–5.

Edelmann, R. and Connolly, K. J. (1986). Psychological Aspects of Infertility. *British Journal of Medical Psychology*, **59**, 209–19.

Edelmann, R. J., Connolly, K. J., Cooke, I. D. and Robson, J. (1991). Psychogenic infertility: some findings. *Journal of Psychosomatic Obstetrics and Gynaecology*, **12**, 163–8.

Edelmann, R. J. and Golombok, S. (1989). Stress and Reproductive Failure. *Journal of Reproductive and Infant Psychology*, **7**, 79–86.

Feuerstein, M., Labbe, E. E. and Kuczmierczyk, A. R. (1986). *Health Psychology: A Psychobiological Perspective*. New York: Plenum Press.

Folkman, S. (1984). Personal Control and Stress and Coping Processes: A Theoretical Analysis. *Journal of Personality and Social Psychology*, **46**, (4), 839–52.

Folkman, S. and Lazarus, R. S. (1980). An Analysis of Coping in a Middle-Aged Community Sample. *Journal of Health and Social Behaviour*, **21**, 219–39.

Folkman, S., Lazarus, R. S., Dunkel-Schetter, C., Delongis, A. and Gruen, R. J. (1986). Dynamics of a stressful encounter: Cognitive appraisal, coping and encounter outcomes. *Journal of Personality and Social Psychology*, **50**, 571–9.

Freeman, E. W., Boxer, A. S., Rickels, K., Tureck, R. and Mastroianni, L. (1985). Psychological evaluation and support in a program of in vitro fertilization and embryo transfer. *Fertility and Sterility*, **43**, (1), 48–53.

Greenglass, E. R. (1982). A world of difference: Gender Role in perspective. Toronto: John Wiley.

Hudson, W. W. and Glisson, D. H. (1982). The clinical measurement package. Homewood, II: Dorsey.

Hull, M. G. R. (1992). The Causes of Infertility and Relative Effectiveness of Treatment. In *Infertility* (A. A. Templeton and J. O. Drife, eds). New York, Springer-Verlag.

Kedem, P., Mikulinger, M. and Nathanson, Y. E. (1990). Psychological aspects of male infertility. *British Journal of Medical Psychology*, **63**, 73–80.

Kraft, A. D., Palombo, J. and Mitchell, D. (1980). The psychological dimensions of infertility. *American Journal of Orthopsychiatry*, **50**, (4), 618–28.

Lalos, A., Lalos, D., Jacobsonn, L. and Schultz, Bo von (1985). The psychological impact of infertility two years after completed surgical treatment. *Obstetrica Gynecologia Scandinavia*, **64**, 599–604.

Link, P. W. and Darling, C. A. (1986). Couples Undergoing Treatment for Infertility: Dimensions of Life Satisfaction. *Journal of Sex and Marital Therapy*, **12**, (1), 46–59.

Mahlstedt, P. (1985). The Psychological Component of Infertility. *Fertility and Sterility*, **43**, (3), 335–47.

Mahlstedt, P. P., Macduff, S. and Bernstein, J. (1987). Emotional Factors and the In-Vitro Fertilization and Embryo Transfer Process. *Journal of In-Vitro Fertilization and Embryo Transfer*, **4**, (4), 232–6.

Mazor, M. D. (1984). Emotional reactions to infertility. In *Infertility: medical, emotional and social considerations* (M. D. Mazor and H. F. Simons, eds). New York: Human Sciences Press.

McGrade, J. J. and Tolor, A. (1981). The reaction to infertility and the infertility investigations: A comparison of the responses of men and women. *Infertility*, **4**, 7–27.

Menning, B. E. (1980). The emotional needs of infertile couples. *Fertility and Sterility*, **34**, 313–19.

Miall, C. E. (1985). Perceptions of Informal Sanctioning and the Stigma of Involuntary Childlessness. *Deviant Behaviour*, **6**, 383–403.

Moller, A. and Fallstrom, K. (1991). Psychological factors in the etiology of infertility: a longitudinal study. *Journal of Psychosomatic Obstetrics and Gynaecology*, **12**, 13–26.

Moos, R. H. and Schaefer, J. A. (1986). Life transitions and crisis: A conceptual overview. In *Coping with Life Crises: An Integrated Approach* (R. Moos, ed.). New York: Plenum Press.

Muller, H. (1985). Human in-vitro fertilization and embryo transfer: expectations and concerns. *Experientia*, **41**, (12), 1515–17.

Paulson, J. D., Haarmann, B. S., Salerno, R. L. and Asmar, P. (1988). An investigation of the relationship between emotional maladjustment and infertility. *Fertility and Sterility*, **49**, (2), 258–62.

Paulson, R. J. and Sauer, M. V. (1991). Counselling the infertile couple when enough is enough. *Obstetrics and Gynaecology*, **78**, 462–4.

Pesch, U., Weyer, G. and Taubert, H. D. (1989). Coping mechanisms in infertile women with luteal phase insufficiency. *Journal of Psychosomatic Obstetrics and Gynaecology*, **10**, 15–23.

Pfeffer, N. and Woollett, A. (1983). *The Experience of Infertility*. London: Virago.

Platt, J. J., Ficher, I. and Silver, M. J. (1973). Infertile couples: Personality traits and self-denial concept discrepancies. *Fertility and Sterility*, **24**, 972–6.

Raval, H., Slade, P., Buck, P. and Lieberman, B. E. (1987). The Impact of Infertility on Emotions and the Marital and Sexual Relationship. *Journal of Reproduction and Infant Psychology*, **5**, 221–34.

Reading, A. E. (1991). Psychological intervention and infertility. In *Infertility: Perspectives from Stress and Coping Research* (A. L. Stanton and C. Dunkel-Schetter, eds). New York: Plenum Press.

Rosenfeld, D. L. and Mitchell, E. (1979). Treating the emotional aspects of infertility: counselling services in an infertility clinic. *American Journal of Obstetrics and Gynaecology*, **135**, (2), 177–80.

Sarason, I. G. and Sarason, B. R. (eds) (1985). *Social Support: Theory, Research and Applications*. Dordrecht: Martinus, Nijhoff.

Seibel, M. and Taymor, M. (1982). Emotional Aspects of Infertility. *Fertility and Sterility*, **37**, (2), 137–45.

Slade, P. (1981). Menstrual cycle symptoms in infertile and control subjects: A re-evaluation of the evidence of psychological changes. *Journal of Psychosomatic Research*, **25**, (3), 175–81.

Stanton, A. L., Tennen, H., Affleck, G. and Mendola, R. (1991). Cognitive Appraisal and Adjustment to Infertility. *Women and Health*, **17**, (3), 1–15.

Stanton, A. L., Tennen, H., Affleck, G. and Mendola, R. (1992). Coping and Adjustment to Infertility. *Journal of Social and Clinical Psychology*, **11**, (1), 1–13.

Strauss, B., Appelt, H., Bohnet, H. G. and Ulrich, D. (1992). Relationship between psychological characteristics and treatment outcome in female patients from an infertility clinic. *Journal of Psychosomatic Obstetrics and Gynaecology*, **13**, 121–133.

Stroebe, N. and Stroebe, M. S. (1987). Bereavement and Health: The Psychological and Physical Consequences of Partner Loss. Cambridge University Press.

Takefman, J. E., Brender, W., Boivin, J. and Tulandi, T. (1990). Sexual and emotional adjustment of couples undergoing infertility investigation and the effectiveness of preparatory information. *Journal of Psychosomatic Obstetrics and Gynaecology*, **11**, 275–90.

Templeton, A. A. (1992). The Epidemiology of Infertility. In *Infertility* (A. A. Templeton and J. O. Drife, eds). New York, Springer-Verlag.

Templeton, A. A., Fraser, C. and Thompson, B. (1991). Infertility – Epidemiology and Referral Practice. *Human Reproduction*, **6**, 1391.

Van Zyl, J. A. (1987). Sex and infertility. Part 1: Prevalence of psychosexual problems and subjacent factors. *South African Medical Journal*, **72**, (7), 482–4.

Veevers, J. E. (1980). Childless by Choice. Toronto: Butterworths.

3

Psychological aspects of the new reproductive technologies

Robert Edelmann and Kevin Connolly

For couples experiencing fertility problems, discussed in Chapter 2, artificial insemination by donor is probably an ancient, 'low tech', technique, practised since the role of sperm in reproduction has been recognized. In contrast the new reproductive technologies involving IVF and surrogacy are revolutionary and 'hi tech' in the extreme. In this chapter Robert Edelmann and Kevin Connolly discuss the psychological implications of these techniques for parents and their offspring, highlighting the secrecy which surrounds some of them and the stress involved in others. As in a number of chapters in this book, they utilize the cognitive appraisal model of stress and coping to provide a theoretical basis for the consideration of stress, coping and intervention.

Introduction

The previous chapter suggested that infertility occurs in around 15% of couples. Some studies have placed the incidencies higher, a pilot study in the UK finding that between 20 and 35% of couples take more than one year to conceive at some point in their reproductive history (Page, 1989), and a regional investigation finding that one in eight childless couples seek specialist advice in their efforts to conceive (Hull, Galzener, Kelly et al., 1985). Infertility is usually defined as a failure to conceive after one year of regular sexual intercourse without the use of contraception (Benson, 1983). Although many couples who experience difficulties will eventually conceive by natural means, many embark upon prolonged investigation and treatment in the hope of satisfying their desire for children. As medical technology has advanced, so the demand for services has increased. Snowden and Snowden (1984) estimated that by the end of the 1970s about 2000 children in Britain and 15 000 in the USA were born annually as a result of donor insemination (DI). These figures are now almost certainly exceeded. Between 1978, when the first successful outcome of in-vitro fertilization (IVF) was achieved, and 1990, more than 5000 infants were born world-wide as a result of this procedure (Cook, 1990). In addition, many hundreds of children are known to have been born in the USA through surrogacy arrangements (Bartels, 1990). The number of such children born in the UK is unknown although some specific cases have been well documented and actual live births are thought to exceed 100.

The most straightforward of these reproductive procedures is undoubtedly DI. DI is considered in cases of male sterility such as azoospermia (absence of sperm) or oligospermia (few sperm) or those involving rhesus (Rh) incompatibility or hereditary disease such as Huntingdon's chorea. However, while the general procedure itself is simple enough, the associated psychological issues encountered by the couple are likely to be complex. These include the couple's adaptation to a child produced by donor insemination and the secrecy which is usually associated with this means of producing a family (Edelmann, 1989).

IVF is an altogether more complex and physically demanding procedure. Although aspects of treatment vary between clinics, it can often involve about a week of outpatient monitoring by the daily estimation of plasma 17-beta-oestradil levels, the daily scoring of cervical mucus, and one or two ovarian ultrasound examinations. This is then followed by a further week of inpatient care, involving frequent hormonal assays, the laparoscopic collection of oocytes and, in the case of successful oocyte collection and fertilization, the embryo transfer (Woods and Trounson, 1982). Unfortunately, success rates for IVF are relatively low with figures between 12 and 20% per cycle being the norm. A world-wide assessment of 50 IVF programmes revealed a 13% success rate per IVF cycle (Soules, 1985). The low success rate has important implications in that the majority of couples entering an IVF programme may be vulnerable to psychological problems not just as a result of the stress involved in the procedure but also as a consequence of their failure to conceive (Edelmann, 1990).

Surrogacy arrangements generally involve either the technically straightforward DI or the technically more complex IVF procedures. DI surrogacy involves a man who is able to produce fertile semen, his partner, who is unable for genetic or physical reasons to provide an oocyte, and a third party who is inseminated with the male's sperm and who then acts as a host, carrying the child to term. IVF surrogacy also involves a host who carries a child for a couple, but in this instance both the oocyte and semen are provided by the couple who wish to have a child. In the former case the resulting child is genetically related to the host, in the latter this is not so. Two instances of DI surrogacy, one in the USA and one in the UK have been widely publicized; in the US case because the host changed her mind about handing the child to its biological father and his partner (Bartels, Priester, Vawter and Caplan, 1990) and in the UK case because of a decision taken by health care workers to take the new born child into care and the subsequent 'kidnap' of the child from a hospital by his biological father (Cotton, 1992). Such issues have led to constraints on the practice of officially sanctioned (i.e. hospital-based) DI surrogacy in the UK and concerns about psychological issues in respect of IVF surrogacy (Edelmann and Connolly, 1994).

In each of these three areas there is some overlapping relation to psychological factors that have been investigated (Edelmann and Connolly, 1994). These relate to the psychological characteristics of individuals and couples involved in the procedure (both the recipients and donors/surrogates), the impact of the procedure itself on the couples concerned and their counselling needs. In the case of DI a further issue relates to the secrecy which normally surrounds the procedure and the psychological consequences for the children brought up in ignorance of their origin. These issues are addressed in this chapter.

Donor insemination

DI is the treatment of choice in relation to male infertility though in effect it by-passes rather than treats the male partner. The procedure requires the woman, who is not directly implicated in the cause of the problem, to monitor her menstrual cycle to determine her fertile period and attend for insemination. If fresh semen is used, the timing of semen collection must be coordinated with the recipient's ovulation. Until the 1970s fresh semen was generally used but given the need to test and retest donors for sexually transmitted diseases and, in particular, acquired immune deficiency syndrome (AIDS) the exclusive use of frozen semen seems likely in the future. The overall success rate with both frozen and fresh semen is about 75% although more cycles seem to be necessary to achieve conception with frozen semen.

Although the emotional impact of infertility diagnosis and treatment has been well documented, couples entering a DI programme, as with others seeking infertility treatment, tend to be well adjusted. The assessment of a consecutive series of 60 women admitted to a DI programme revealed a uniformly positive attitude towards the treatment, uniformly high marital adjustment scores and low neuroticism and psychoticism scores in relation to age norms. However, scores on the lie scale were higher (Cox and Reading, 1983; Reading, Sledmere and Cox, 1982). This evidence thus suggests that women attending the DI clinic were calm, controlled individuals who had chosen, in conjunction with their partners, a socially acceptable solution to their problem.

However, concerns about the possible psychological implications of DI for the couples involved have been raised. Because the biological identity of one parent is known beyond doubt, there is a risk of some psychological imbalance being created in the relationship between the natural mother, the social father and the child. This may be a particularly important factor given that recent reports suggest that a diagnosis of male infertility may lead to more distress for the couple than a diagnosis of female infertility (Connolly, Edelmann and Cooke, 1987; Connolly, Edelmann, Cooke and Robson, 1992). The ability to father a child may be seen as confirmation of a man's virility or serve other identity needs (Callan, 1982). Infertility and virility can become confused so that a man who is unable to father a child may feel that others doubt his masculinity (Mahlstedt, 1985). Some have argued that the DI child may serve as a constant reminder to the male of his inadequacy (Clamar, 1981). The empirical data relating to this issue is limited but it lends some support to this view. David and Avidan (1976) in a study of 44 DI couples who were interviewed either before or after conception, or following delivery, report that 80% of husbands felt guilt both about what they saw as their inability to prove their manhood or to act as real fathers and because they felt responsible for their wives having to undergo treatment. Such issues partly explain the widespread preference for secrecy voiced by DI couples and are also likely to have significant implications for counselling.

Counselling and donor insemination

The Warnock Committee's (1984) recommendation that in Britain DI should be confined to centres with trained counsellors recognizes the complex emotional issues surrounding decisions that couples make with regard to DI (DHSS, 1984). Ideally, counselling should facilitate the couple's decision-making, helping some to acknowledge that DI is not an appropriate solution for their childlessness while clarifying for others that it is a means they wish to follow. In this context Menning (1981) argues that, with counselling, couples will effectively screen themselves in or out. Humphrey, Humphrey and Ainsworth-Smith (1991) make an important distinction between screening (that is testing for the presence or absence of a particular quality) and vetting (making a thorough appraisal of suitability). With respect to DI they argue in favour of the former but not the latter. The task of the counsellor or psychologist is not to exclude those who would make inadequate parents, but rather to help those couples for whom DI might generate or exacerbate emotional problems to effectively screen themselves out from the treatment. The question of counselling couples subsequent to DI has rarely been dealt with in the literature. For many the outcome, in terms of conceptions, is likely to be successful and the counselling needs for these are likely to be quite different from those where it fails. The preference for secrecy referred to earlier makes it difficult to ascertain the counselling needs of DI families.

Secrecy and donor insemination

A number of reports document the widespread preference for secrecy voiced by DI couples. From a telephone and mail survey of 427 women who had conceived by DI during the previous 12 years, 61% indicated they probably or definitely would not tell their children about their mode of conception, 18% said they probably or definitely would and 21% were undecided (Amuzu, Loxava and Shapiro, 1990). Clayton and Kovacs (1982) in a survey of 50 Australian couples some two to four years after donor insemination, report that 68% had decided they would definitely not tell their child of its origins. Eighteen per cent were undecided and only 14% had made up their minds to tell their child at some later date. These figures are not markedly dissimilar to those reported with similar samples in other cultures. Manuel, Chevret and Czyba (1980) found that 77% of 72 DI couples in a French series preferred absolute secrecy while Owens, Edelmann and Humphrey (1993) found that 74% of 76 couples with male infertility had no intention of telling a child conceived through DI about the mode of conception. Rowland (1985) in a further study in the UK found that 56% of couples had already decided before undertaking DI that they would definitely not tell their child about its origins. In this latter study, 9% of couples had decided they would tell their child and 36% remained undecided, suggesting that the figures would eventually come to closely resemble those reported by Clayton and Kovacs. Even among clinicians there is a tendency to favour non-disclosure, Leiblum and Hamkins (1992) reporting a survey of 364 reproductive endo-crinologists revealed that 56% favoured non-disclosure, 22% felt that children should be told and 21% endorsed a neutral viewpoint. One per cent of the sample did not respond.

It has been suggested (e.g. Snowden, Mitchell and Snowden, 1983) that secrecy is designed to protect the couple and more especially the male partner. However, there is an obvious question concerning whether the child has a right to know of the nature of his/her conception. Secrecy deprives the child of this right. We also have little information about the extent to which secrecy might be harmful for either the child and/or the family in which the child is raised. Reports tend to suggest a relatively favourable outcome from DI in terms of paternal involvement in childrearing and a low incidence of divorce. However, there are few reliable figures and the attendant secrecy makes such matters very difficult to investigate. Family relationships run the risk of being seriously damaged when they are based on deception, and such deceptions lead to stress and anxiety (Menning, 1981). In addition, there is an ever present danger that the child may learn the truth by accident with potentially very damaging repercussions. Given such dangers it seems reasonable to conclude that openness concerning DI should be encouraged. The information that is available, though extremely limited, suggests that DI children told of their origin are not harmed by such disclosure (Daniels and Taylor, 1993). However, the question of whether a DI child should be told, and if so how, when and with what kind of message is inevitably a difficult question to answer (see Daniels and Taylor, 1993 and the accompanying commentaries for a full discussion of the issues involved).

Motivation of semen donors

Secrecy not only raises issues for the children conceived by DI and their families but also for semen donors (Daniels, 1989). It is generally presumed that donors should be protected from unwanted contact from any child who is a product of the donation and that just as the child should not know the identity of the donor, so the donor should not know of the child's existence. The secrecy/anonymity that has surrounded donor insemination inevitably means that little research has been conducted to date examining motives and attitudes of semen donors. In one small-scale study of 23 semen donors in Australia, Daniels (1989) reported that 20 (91%) of the men cited a desire to help infertile couples as their reason for donating semen (an identical percentage was obtained in an earlier small-scale study of 37 semen donors in New Zealand; Daniels, 1987). Eighteen of the men (82%) stated that anonymity was either important or very important to them (the comparable figure reported by Daniels from New Zealand was 95%). Interestingly 11 (50%) felt that the child should be able to discover the identity of the donor while 16 (73%) stated that they would still donate semen even if their offspring could trace them (the comparable figures reported by Daniels in 1987 were 16% and 24% respectively).

In-vitro fertilization

As with DI, it seems that couples presenting for IVF are generally well adjusted and in stable relationships. A number of studies have administered psychological tests to patients admitted into IVF programmes and have found little difference between scores obtained by these couples and the normative test data or data from appropriate comparison groups (see Edelmann, 1990). Two investigations studies will serve as examples. Newton, Hearn and Yuzpe (1990) found that group means from a very large sample of IVF couples (947 women and 899 men) were well within the clinically normal range three months before the first IVF attempt. Edelmann, Connolly and Bartlett (1994) examined 150 couples, who were consecutive referrals for their first IVF cycle, and found little evidence of variation from the normative range on a number of psychological measures.

The only exception to these findings is the occasional report of elevated anxiety in women attending IVF clinics (e.g. Cook, Parsons, Mason and Golombok, 1989; Johnston, Shaw and Bird, 1987). This is likely to be associated with clinic attendance itself rather than reflecting a particular feature of IVF treatment and as such is not surprising. As our own findings indicate, elevated anxiety is found before diagnosis and when the couple first attend a specialist clinic. This declines subsequently in spite of numerous potentially distressing investigative procedures and several possible diagnostic outcomes which are less than positive (Connolly, Edelmann, Cooke and Robson, 1992). Indeed, as Johnston, Shaw and Bird (1987) note, the anxiety levels of their IVF couples were similar to data obtained by their colleagues from women attending an antenatal clinic during the final two weeks of their pregnancy. Overall there is no evidence to support the view that couples electing for IVF differ systematically from couples conceiving children by natural means. Indeed, it is possible that only those with a stable disposition and who enjoy stable relationships decide to proceed with IVF and hence submit themselves to the inevitable stressors associated with the procedure.

The stressful nature of IVF

Clinic attendance

A number of authors (e.g. Leiblum, Kemmann and Lane, 1987) have commented on the great emotional strain placed upon couples undergoing IVF. The IVF cycle lasts about two weeks, and involves about one week of outpatient monitoring and one week of clinic care, though aspects of the programme may vary considerably between clinics. Because there is a risk of failure at any of the stages of the IVF procedure, each cycle of IVF has many potential points likely to create anxiety and lead to distress. These include concerns about the fertilization process, fear of laparoscopy, pressures on the male to produce a semen sample on demand, anxiety at the time of embryo transfer and the results of pregnancy tests (Greenfeld and Haseltine, 1986). Such concerns and anxieties have been documented in a number of studies (e.g. Connolly, Edelmann, Bartlett et al., 1993).

In a study by Callan and Hennessey (1986) the majority of the 77 women undergoing IVF who were interviewed associated some anxiety with each stage of the programme. The most anxiety provoking episodes were during the initial waiting at home, in hospital just prior to egg collection and during surgery for egg collection. This latter phase was also found to be associated with heightened anxiety by Johnston, Shaw and Bird (1987), who also found that the first visit to the IVF assessment clinic was a time of particularly heightened anxiety. A general trend towards increasing stress and distress during the IVF treatment cycle was reported by Reading, Chang and Kerin (1989), although overall scores remained low compared with normative data. It is interesting that these authors also note that greater distress (as measured by an index of grief) was apparent for women who discontinued treatment at midcycle compared with those who completed the cycle even if they failed to achieve a pregnancy. Indeed, there is general agreement among studies that the time waiting to hear if fertilization has occurred and to hear the results after embryo transfer are the procedures and stages of the IVF process that couples find most stressful (Baram, Tourtelot, Muechler and Huan, 1988; Connolly, Edelmann, Bartlett et al., 1993; Laffont and Edelmann, 1994; Seibel and Levine, 1987). These are clearly key points in the IVF process and occur at times when the patient has little control over events and little contact with, and hence support from, the medical team.

In addition to anxiety provoked by the procedure itself some authors have suggested that anxiety can vary over repeated treatment cycles although the only empirical investigation to address this issue (Reading, Chang and Kerin, 1989) found no significant effects of repeated treatment on psychological state. These results were, however, based upon a small sample ($N = 37$).

Stress and success rates for IVF

Success rates from IVF are relatively low and yet couples entering IVF treatment programmes tend to be over optimistic about their own chances of success (Johnston, Shaw and Bird, 1987; Reading, 1989). In the former series, all the patients overestimated the likelihood of success, however such optimism is unlikely to be peculiar to those attending IVF clinics. The authors relate their findings to evidence that denial and avoidance are used successfully as coping strategies by surgical patients generally. Overestimation may thus serve to reduce the stress associated with the procedure.

The emotional strain imposed by IVF has important practical implications, both for counselling provision, and because of its potential effects on the menstrual cycle and ovulation. While the low success rates are perhaps largely attributable to procedural and biomedical factors it is plausible to assume that psychological stressors may also serve to reduce success rates via effects on the neuroendocrine system. Indeed, in one study (Thiering, Beaurepaire, Jones et al., 1993), follow-up 12 months after initial assessment, and after controlling for number of treatment cycles, indicated a significantly lower pregnancy rate in depressed compared to non-depressed women. It is also reasonable to assume that fertility of the male involved in the procedure will also be influenced by the stresses imposed by IVF. Harrison, Callan and Hennessey (1987) compared semen samples collected in the couple's pre-IVF workup with a second sample collected some five weeks later to inseminate the eggs in-vitro (specific stress measures were not taken). Although for 91% of the 500 cases there was no change between successive samples in the assigned fertility index, 35 cases (7%) showed a change in classification from normal to pathologic or severely pathologic categories. For these cases the incidence of total fertilization failure in the procedure increased dramatically. Although the authors assume that the change was provoked by emotional stress, it is necessary, as they point out, to test the assumption by including appropriate measures of stress in the assessment procedure.

Unsuccessful IVF

The emotional impact of unsuccessful IVF has been examined in a number of studies many of which refer to feelings of sadness, anger and depression, particularly in the case of women. Leiblum, Kemmann and Lane (1987) reported that wives were significantly more depressed, guilty, angry, 'empty' and sad than their husbands following unsuccessful IVF. Greater severity of depression for women compared with men following IVF failure has been reported by Baram, Tourtelot, Muechler and Huan (1988). Newton, Hearn and Yuzpe (1990) found increases in anxiety and depression for both men and women following a failed first cycle of IVF with the prevalence of both mild and moderate depression increasing substantially, particularly among women. Given the circumstances it would probably be unusual if such reactions were other than the norm for the couples concerned.

In-vitro fertilization treatment is undeniably stressful for the couple concerned and sadness or depression would be neither unexpected or unusual reactions to failed attempts. Most couples embarking on IVF are emotionally well adjusted and in stable relationships; consequently, they probably have the coping resources needed to enable them to deal with the emotional demands involved.

Coping and IVF

In a study of 155 couples who were consecutive referrals to an IVF clinic the most commonly endorsed coping strategy used by both men and women was direct action (Edelmann, Connolly and Bartlett, 1994). This is perhaps not surprising since it is consistent with their behaviour (i.e. taking action by seeking treatment to resolve their infertility). Whether the decision to take direct action serves to make a couple psychologically vulnerable in the event of IVF failure is a matter of interest. In the case of women, in our own study, direct action only seemed to be positively related to well being if it was associated with some degree of acceptance of one's position: that is accepting that the problem is inevitable and that nothing can be done about it. For men, the picture was less clear; while direct action and acceptance appeared to be positive coping strategies, a redefinition of the situation, that is trying to see the problem in a different light which makes it seem more bearable, also seemed to play an important role.

A few other studies have also examined the effect of coping strategy upon adjustment to IVF treatment or to the failure of treatment. The findings support the notion that active or problem-focused coping serves a protective function in contrast to avoidance coping. Thus, in a study of 40 women attending for IVF treatment, Demyttenaere, Nijs, Evers-Kiebooms and Koninckx (1991) found that active coping was associated with a tendency to be less easily depressed. In a study of 36 couples who failed to conceive as a result of IVF, Litt, Tennen, Affleck and Klock (1992) found that women who employed more escape coping before IVF were more distressed by its failure. In a further study of 100 women progressing through a treatment cycle, Hynes, Callan, Terry and Gallois (1992) found that use of problem-focused coping was associated with high levels of post-attempt well-being, while the use of avoidance coping and seeking social support was associated with low levels of well being. The strong evidence for the deleterious consequences of avoidance coping is a finding common in studies of individuals coping with chronic illness. Avoidance may be a problem for a number of reasons; it may impede the person's ability to confront and deal with their emotions; it may lead to reliance on inappropriate forms of coping (e.g. drinking alcohol); and attempts to avoid reminders of infertility may lead to a restriction of daily activities (Stanton, 1991). This suggests that one role for counselling might be to promote a positive reappraisal of the situation and discourage avoidance.

Counselling and IVF

In the UK it has been decided that all centres offering licensed treatment should make counselling available to all couples who are considering such treatment (DHSS, 1987). However, both the type of counselling provided and its availability vary widely from clinic to clinic. For example, counselling has been interpreted by some as implying the need to provide information and by others as implying the provision of an opportunity for couples to talk through their concerns. While counselling in some form should be available, this does not imply that all couples will make use of it. In a sample of over 100 couples presenting for IVF, Laffont and Edelmann (1994) found that three-quarters expressed a wish for a meeting with a psychologist prior to treatment and almost half the sample expressed a wish for such support during the course of treatment. Similarly, Shaw, Johnston and Shaw (1987) report that half their sample of 60 couples awaiting IVF treatment requested counselling. Lower figures are reported by Baram, Tourtelot, Muechler and Huan (1988). In their study only 24% of women and 13% of men in the sample felt that long-term counselling would have been helpful following the failure of IVF. Cultural differences in the meaning attributed to psychological and counselling support, the differences in the way in which questions were phrased, and the methods used in these studies no doubt partly explain the variations in results. Suffice to say that many couples would welcome the provision of counselling although there is limited information available on the many issues which arise concerning the provision of counselling. These include discovering the forms of support which are most needed and which couples might benefit most from counselling.

The one study to date evaluating counselling provision suggests that in many cases counselling may not convey any benefits additional to the provision of clear information about the treatment process (Connolly Edelmann, Bartlett et al., 1993). In this study, 155 couples who were consecutive referrals to an IVF clinic were allocated at random to one of two groups. One group (the control) were given details of the procedures involved in the treatment, and the importance of blood and semen samples was carefully explained. A second (treatment) group was treated in exactly the same way but with the addition of three counselling sessions. These were arranged for the first clinic visit, at the start of the treatment cycle and after either treatment failure or successful conception. The results showed the patients to be generally well adjusted with anxiety levels dropping over the course of treatment. Counselling compared to information alone did not lead to any enhanced reduction in levels of anxiety or depression. The nature and extent of counselling support needed by patients undergoing IVF may be quite modest and may be most appropriate for a subset of vulnerable individuals. The challenge for future research is to identify, first, when that support should be provided, and second, which, probably small, proportion of patients might actually need and benefit from such specialized support. The results of one study do suggest that more distressed women actually felt they would benefit from some form of support (Laffont and Edelmann, 1994).

Surrogacy

Surrogacy generally involves either DI or IVF procedures; in the former case the host is genetically related to the child while in the latter case she is not. Arrangements for DI surrogacy are frequently made privately between the parties concerned and it is therefore difficult to estimate either the number of children born through such procedures or the nature and severity of the psychological problems which may arise. IVF surrogacy arrangements obviously necessitate medical involvement and psychologists and other mental health professionals, particularly in the USA, are asked to screen and counsel both couples seeking surrogacy arrangements and women volunteering to become surrogate mothers (Franks, 1981; Slovenko, 1985). As with semen donors the motivation of women who act as surrogates is most frequently said to be altruistic, for example, the wish to give 'the gift of a baby to a parent who needed a child' (Parker, 1983).

Given that at present we know very little about the consequences of surrogacy, the most important role of assessment is to anticipate what the reactions and responses of those involved might be (Harrison, 1990). The main aims are to judge whether problems are likely to arise in the relationship between the donor couple and host and to judge whether the host will feel able to part with the child after the birth. Harrison suggests that the following main considerations should be addressed in any psychological assessment of surrogates:

- their motivation
- previous conception/childbearing history
- family support
- the task of separating from the child
- the relationship with the donor couple, and
- their views on important matters relating to medical tests and contact between partners during and after a pregnancy.

Although problems cannot be eliminated, careful assessment and counselling should help to reduce the number of difficulties which arise and perhaps ensure that for the most part they are of the kind that can be solved.

Psychological research to date in this area is very limited and a range of issues relating to the parents, host and children remain to be addressed. If such procedures become more common in the future then we clearly need to know more about the motives of hosts, why problems occur and how best to tackle these through counselling, and subsequent reactions of families and their children.

Conclusion

The last decade has seen a steady increase in research relating to psychological aspects of the reproductive technologies. Although this has led to a clearer understanding of the issues involved there are nevertheless substantial gaps in our knowledge as well as a number of contradictory research findings. Perhaps the most robust finding is that couples presenting for infertility treatment are in general psychologically well adjusted and tend to be in stable relationships. This may reflect a process of self-selection in that only those couples who are well adjusted individuals and in stable relationships get as far as seeking specialist medical help in dealing with their failure to have children. It would be difficult to argue, however, that the usually lengthy process of investigation and treatment associated with infertility does not provoke some distress and anxiety. These are normal reactions from well adjusted people exposed to stressful circumstances. IVF in particular is likely to place the couple under a tremendous emotional strain particularly at times of heightened uncertainty, for example, when they are waiting to hear if fertilization has occurred and again when they are waiting for the results following embryo transfer. The emotional impact of unsuccessful IVF has also been considered in a number of studies. In this context, the provision of counselling could help couples cope with emotional difficulties although to date there is little research which addresses the many issues that arise concerning the provision of counselling.

DI is also not without its stresses. In the minds of some the capacity to father a child is seen as confirmation of a man's virility; any man who is unable to father a child may feel that others doubt his masculinity. This may explain research findings which suggest that a diagnosis of male infertility may be more distressing for the couple concerned than a diagnosis of female infertility. It may also explain the tendency for DI parents to opt to maintain secrecy about their child's mode of conception. Unfortunately, little information exists about the extent to which secrecy might be harmful for the child and for the family in which the child is raised. However, the preference for secrecy makes if difficult to answer these questions and indeed makes it difficult to ascertain the counselling needs of DI families.

Some form of counselling should be available to all couples who are considering infertility treatment. More difficult questions concern what form such counselling should take, when it should be provided and with what particular aims in mind. Ideally, counselling should facilitate the couple's decision-making process, promote in them a positive reappraisal of their situation and facilitate effective coping. Research is slowly addressing the important issues but with rapid medical advances it is important not to lose sight of the ethical, moral, legal and psychological concerns (Council for Science and Society, 1984).

Applications

1. More research is needed into the effects of DI on children. Given the level of current knowledge, it seems reasonable to suggest that there should be greater openness concerning DI.

2. It needs to be recognized that techniques such as IVF will invariably cause stress and that this is not a reflection of any psychological vulnerability in the couples involved.

3. The counselling needs of couples undergoing IVF seem relatively modest. Evidence to date suggests that counselling might usefully promote positive appraisal and provide support.

Further reading

Stanton, A., Dunkel-Schetter, C. (eds) (1991). *Infertility: Perspectives from Stress and Coping Research*. New York: Plenum Press.
Stanworth, M. (1988). *Reproductive technologies: gender, motherhood and medicine*. Cambridge: Polity Press.

References

Amuzu, B., Loxava, R. and Shapiro, S. (1990). Pregnancy outcome, health of children, and family adjustment after donor insemination. *Obstetrics and Gynecology*, **75**, 899–908.
Baram, D., Tourtelot, E., Meuchler, E. and Huan, K. E. (1988). Psychosocial adjustment following unsuccessful in vitro fertilization. *Journal of Psychosomatic Obstetrics and Gynaecology*, **9**, 181–90.
Bartels, D. M. (1990). Surrogacy arrangements: an overview. In *Beyond Baby M* (D. M. Bartels, P. Preister, D. E. Vawter and A. I. Caplan, eds). Clifton, New Jersey: Humana Press.
Bartels, D. M., Preister, P., Vawter, D. E. and Caplan, A. I. (eds) (1990) *Beyond Baby M*. Clifton, New Jersey: Humana Press.
Benson, R. C. (1983). *Handbook of Obstetrics and Gynecology*. Los Altos, CA; Lange Medical Publishers.
Callan, V. J. (1982). Childlessness and partner selection. *Journal of Marriage and the Family*, **45**, 181–6.
Callan, V. J. and Hennessey, J. F. (1986). IVF and adoption: the experience of infertile couples. *Australian Journal of Early Childhood*, **11**, 32–6.
Clamar, A. (1981). Artificial insemination by donor: the anonymous pregnancy. *American Journal of Forensic Psychology*, **2**, 27–37.
Clayton, C. S. and Kovacs, G. (1982). AID offspring: initial follow-up study of 50 couples. *Medical Journal of Australia*, 338–9.
Connolly, K. J., Edelmann, R. J., Bartlett, H., Cooke, I. D. and Lenton, L. (1993). An evaluation of counselling for couples undergoing treatment for in vitro fertilization. *Human Reproduction*, **8**, 1332–8.
Connolly, K. J., Edelmann, R. J. and Cooke, I. D. (1987). Distress and marital problems associated with infertility. *Journal of Reproductive and Infant Psychology*, **5**, 49–57.
Connolly, K. J., Edelmann, R. J., Cooke, I. D. and Robson, J. (1992). The impact of infertility investigations upon psychological functioning. *Journal of Psychosomatic Research*, **36**, 459–68.
Cook, C. L. (1990). The gynecologic perspective. In *Psychiatric Aspects of Reproductive Technology* (N. L. Stotland, ed.) Washington DC: American Psychiatric Press.
Cook, R., Parsons, J., Mason, S. and Golombok, S. (1989). Emotional, marital and sexual functioning in patients embarking upon IVF and AID treatment for infertility. *Journal of Reproductive and Infant Psychology*, **7**, 87–94.
Cotton, K. (1992). *Second Time Around*. New Barnet, Herts: K. Cotton.
Council for Science and Society (1984). *Human Procreation: Ethical Aspects of the New Techniques*. Oxford: Oxford University Press.
Cox, D. N. and Reading, A. E. (1983). Personality profiles of women attending an artificial insemination by donor clinic. *Personality and Individual Differences*, **4**, 213–4.
Daniels, K. R. (1987). Semen donors in New Zealand: their characteristics and attitudes. *Clinical Reproduction and Fertility*, **5**, 177–90.
Daniels, K. R. (1989). Semen donors: their motivations and attitudes to their offspring. *Journal of Reproductive and Infant Psychology*, **7**, 121–7.
Daniels, K. R. and Taylor, K. (1993). Secrecy and openness in donor insemination. *Politics and the Life Sciences*, **12**, 155–70.
David, A. and Avidan, M. A. (1976). Artificial insemination donor: clinical and psychological aspects. *Fertility and Sterility*, **27**, 528–32.
Demyttenaere, K., Nijs, P., Evers-Kiebooms, G. and Koninckx, P. R. (1991). Coping, ineffectiveness

of coping and the psychoendocrinological stress responses during in vitro fertilisation. *Journal of Psychosomatic Research*, **35**, 231–43.

Department of Health and Social Security (1984). *Human Fertilization and Embryology: A Framework for Legislation*. Cmnd 259, London: HMSO.

Department of Health and Social Security (1987). *Human Fertilization and Embryology*. Report of the Committee Chairman: Dame Mary Warnock DBE. Cmnd 9314, London: HMSO.

Edelmann, R. J. (1983). Psychological evaluation for 'surrogate' motherhood arrangements. Paper presented at the British Psychological Society London Conference, City University.

Edelmann, R. J. (1989). Psychological aspects of artificial insemination by donor. *Journal of Psychosomatic Obstetrics and Gynaecology*, **10**, 3–13.

Edelmann, R. J. (1990). Emotional aspects of in vitro fertilization procedures: a review. *Journal of Reproductive and Infant Psychology*, **8**, 161–73.

Edelmann, R. J. and Connolly, K. J. (1994). Reproductive failure and the reproductive technologies: a psychological perspective. In *Health Psychology: A Lifespan Perspective* (G. Penny, P. Bennett and M. Herbert, eds). London: Harwood Academic Press.

Edelmann, R. J., Connolly, K. J. and Bartlett, H. (1994). Coping strategies and psychological adjustment of couples presenting for IVF. *Journal of Psychosomatic Research*, **38**, 355–64.

Franks, D. D. (1981). Psychiatric evaluation of women in a surrogate mother program. *American Journal of Psychiatry*, **138**, 1378–9.

Greenfeld, D. and Haseltine, F. (1986). Candidate selection and psychosocial considerations of in vitro fertilization procedures. *Clinical Obstetrics and Gynecology*, **29**, 119–26.

Harrison, M. (1990). Psychological ramifications of 'surrogate' motherhood. In *Psychiatric Aspects of Reproductive Technology* (N. L. Stotland, ed.) Washington DC: American Psychiatric Press.

Harrison, K. L., Callan, V. J. and Hennessey, J. F. (1987). Stress and semen quality in an in vitro fertilization program. *Fertility and Sterility*, **48**, 633–6.

Hull, M. G. R., Glazener, C. M. A., Kelly, N. J., Conway, D. J., Foster, P. A., Hinton, R. A., Coulson, C., Lambert, P. A., Watt, E. M. and Desai, K. M. (1985). Population study of causes, treatment and outcome of infertility. *British Medical Journal*, **291**, 1693–7.

Humphrey, M., Humphrey, H. and Ainsworth-Smith, I. (1991). Screening couples for parenthood by donor insemination. *Social Science and Medicine*, **32**, 273–8.

Hynes, G. J., Callan, V. J., Terry, D. J. and Gallois, C. (1992). The psychological well-being of infertile women after a failed IVF attempt: the effects of coping. *British Journal of Medical Psychology*, **65**, 269–78.

Johnston, M., Shaw, R. and Bird, D. (1987). Test-tube baby procedures: stress and judgements under uncertainty. *Psychology and Health*, **1**, 25–38.

Laffont, I. and Edelmann, R. J. (1994). Psychological aspects of in vitro fertilization: a gender comparison. *Journal of Psychosomatic Obstetrics and Gynaecology*, **15**, 22–25.

Leiblum, S. R. and Hamkins, S. E. (1992). To tell or not to tell: attitudes of reproductive endocrinologists concerning disclosure to offspring of conception via assisted insemination by donor. *Journal of Psychosomatic Obstetrics and Gynaecology*, **13**, 267–75.

Leiblum, S. R., Kemmann, E. and Lane, M. K. (1987). The psychological concomitants of in vitro fertilization failure. *Journal of Behavioral Medicine*, **215**, 171–87.

Litt, M. D., Tennen, H., Affleck, G., Klock, S. (1992). Coping and cognitive factors in adaptation to in vitro fertilization failure. *Journal of Behavioral Medicine*, **15**, 171–87.

Mahlstedt, P. P. (1985). The psychological components of infertility. *Fertility and Sterility*, **43**, 335–46.

Manuel, C., Chevret, M. and Czyba, J. C. (1980). Handling of secrecy by DI couples. In *Human Artificial Insemination and Semen Preservation* (G. David and W. S. Price, eds). New York: Plenum Press.

Menning, B. E. (1981). Donor insemination. The psychological issues. *Contemporary Obstetrics and Gynecology*, **18**, 155–72.

Newton, C. R., Hearn, M. T. and Yuzpe, A. A. (1990). Psychological assessment and follow-up after in vitro fertilization: Assessing the impact of failure. *Fertility and Sterility*, **54**, 879–86.

Owens, D. J., Edelmann, R. J. and Humphrey, M. E. (1993). Male infertility and donor insemination: couples' decisions, reactions and counselling needs. *Human Reproduction*, **8**, 880–85.

Page, H. (1989). Estimation of the prevalence and incidence of infertility in a population: a pilot study. *Fertility and Sterility*, **51**, 571–7.

Parker, P. J. (1983). Motivation of surrogate mothers: initial findings. *American Journal of Psychiatry*, **140**, 117–18.

Reading, A. E. (1989). Decision making and in vitro fertilization: the influence of emotional states. *Journal of Psychosomatic Obstetrics and Gynaecology*, **10**, 107–12.

Reading, A. E., Chang, L. C. and Kerin, J. F. (1989). Psychological state and coping styles across an IVF treatment cycle. *Journal of Reproductive and Infant Psychology*, **7**, 95–103.

Reading, A. E., Sledmere, C. M. and Cox, D. N. (1982). A survey of patients' attitudes towards artificial insemination by donor. *Journal of Psychosomatic Research*, **26**, 429–33.

Rowland, R. (1985). The social and psychological consequences of secrecy in artificial insemination by donor. *Social Science and Medicine*, **21**, 391–6.

Seibel, M. M. and Levine, S. (1987). A new era of reproduction technologies: the emotional stages of in vitro fertilization. *Journal of In Vitro Fertilization and Embryo Transfer*, **4**, 135–40.

Shaw, P., Johnston, M. and Shaw, R. (1987). Counselling needs, emotional and relationship problems in couples awaiting IVF. *Journal of Psychosomatic Obstetrics and Gynaecology*, **9**, 171–80.

Slovenko, R. (1985). Obstetric science and the developing role of the psychiatrist in surrogate motherhood. *Journal of Psychiatry and Law*, **13**, 487–518.

Snowden, R., Mitchell, G. D. and Snowden, E. M. (1983). *Artificial Reproduction: A Social Investigation*. London: Allen and Unwin.

Snowden, R. and Snowden, E. (1984). *The Gift of a Child*. London: Allen and Unwin.

Soules, M. R. (1985). The in vitro fertilization rate: let's be honest with one another. *Fertility and Sterility*, **43**, 511–13.

Stanton, A. L. (1991). Cognitive appraisals, coping processes and adjustment to infertility. In *Infertility: Perspectives from Stress and Coping Research* (A. L. Stanton and C. Dunkel-Schetter, eds). New York: Plenum Press.

Thiering, P., Beaurepaire, J., Jones, M., Saunders, D. and Tennant, C. (1993). Mood state as a predictor of treatment outcome after in vitro fertilization/embryo transfer technology (IVF/ET). *Journal of Psychosomatic Research*, **37**, 481–91.

Woods, C. and Trounson, A. O. (1982). In vitro fertilization and embryo transfer. In *Recent Advances in Obstetrics and Gynaecology* (J. Bonner, ed.). London: Churchill Livingstone.

4

Pregnancy: a bio-psycho-social event

Gill Scott and Catherine Niven

> The chapter sets the scene for the remainder of the book in dealing with the range of events and experiences which can follow conception. In this chapter Gill Scott and Catherine Niven view pregnancy from a bio-psycho-social perspective, reflecting the theoretical theme of the book series. As in Chapter 3, the cognitive appraisal model of stress is utilized, in this case to bring together the biological, psychological and social aspects of stress in pregnancy and to examine the ways in which society, and its microcosm the family, can provide the necessary resources to ameliorate its effects.

Pregnancy can be considered from separate biological, psychological and sociological perspectives. However this chapter will argue that it is best encapsulated in a bio-psycho-social framework. Pregnancy/gestation in mammals is the period from conception to delivery of offspring when successful, and thus represents a biological event of great importance. In humans, pregnancy is a long drawn out event the status of which is uncertain for some time after conception. While these biological realities of pregnancy are unchanging, social, pharmacological and medical developments have altered the experience of pregnancy for women in different generations.

The changing experience of pregnancy

The last one hundred years have seen massive changes in pregnancy – how it is experienced by women, its outcomes, the level of medical intervention and the level of social control and support exercised over it. Not least among these changes is the number of pregnancies women experience. The dramatic decrease of time spent pregnant by women is highlighted if we compare the contemporary average of three years of a woman's life in the UK spent pregnant (Oakley, 1993) with a personal account collected by Llewelyn Davies (1978) in the early part of this century: 'For fifteen years I was in a very poor state of health owing to continual pregnancy. As soon as I was over one trouble it was all started over again.'

A major factor related to this decrease is that women can now control their fertility and they expect pregnancy to result in a healthy child with a high life expectancy. There is little doubt that childbirth has become much safer as well as much less frequent for women in contemporary industrial societies. For example in England and Wales in 1925–30 the maternal mortality rate was 4.7 per thousand live births. By 1980 this had fallen to 0.12 per thousand (Dally, 1982). This is a picture repeated throughout the industrialized world, although with slight differences in rates and times (Loudon, 1992a).

Besides changes in the number and rate of success of pregnancies in industrial societies there have also been major changes in the social organization of obstetric care. Such changes, however, are not always positive (Halinka Maloe, 1994). Indeed between 1870 and 1930 in England and Wales, maternal mortality was often higher in the middle and upper classes than in the working classes and, according to Loudon (1992b) it was greater use of medical obstetrics by the middle classes that explained the difference. Obstetric care is much safer now, but recent changes in medical techniques to enable conception, to screen the fetus and to monitor the health of the mother-to-be continue to affect the physical experience of pregnancy. Pregnancy may now involve frequent contact with health practitioners and exposure to a range of physical experiences ranging in invasiveness from ultrasound to embryo transfer.

A final way in which pregnancy has changed is in its social context. The way in which a society responds to pregnancy seriously affects the psychological and material, as well as the biological, well being of women. Key factors here are attitudes towards pregnancy, family structures and systems of welfare for pregnant women. Attitudes to pregnancy and the treatment of pregnant women vary from society to society. For example in Victorian Britain and in some modern day Islamic societies pregnancy is regarded as a source of embarrassment because of its association with sexuality and is kept a secret for as long as possible. This can have implications for health care which may not be provided until late in pregnancy or if available may not be utilized (Currer, 1986; Morse, 1989). In other societies where concepts of health reflect an emphasis on kinship, sharing and community, for example in native Fijian society, pregnancy is a community event and the health of the pregnant woman is the concern of the entire community, even the children (Morse, 1989). By contrast in societies where the profession of medicine has greater control over concepts of health, pregnancy has become medicalized (Oakley, 1984). Such changes have had a powerful influence on attitudes towards pregnancy and on the way the pregnant woman is cared for, with the result that women's own perceptions of pregnancy are often overlooked (Graham and Oakley, 1986).

These changes may have a powerful effect on the psychological experience of pregnancy, but one further area of change affecting pregnancy over the last few decades is that of social policy. Material as well as social and psychological forms of support for pregnant women have changed significantly. Employment legislation, maternity benefits, state medical care and welfare support during pregnancy can ease the material demands that women experience in the later stages of pregnancy. However, these are not always developed neutrally. Lewis (1980) argues that maternal welfare policies during this century have often been a hidden cover for an extensive public regulation of motherhood and social reproduction. For example, pregnant women in France are required to attend antenatal clinics at regular intervals in order to receive state benefits. Another example of conditional support is provided by Ni and Rossignol's study of maternal mortality in the Sichuan province of China between 1989 and 1991. They argue that the higher mortality rates amongst mothers with unplanned pregnancies resulted from China's one child policy. The negative economic sanctions endured by women who ignored the policy (loss of wages, loss of free prenatal care) as well as the anxiety and isolation of the mothers, are cited as reasons for their higher rate of pregnancy complications and maternal mortality (Ni and Rossignol, 1994).

The experience of pregnancy today then differs considerably from that of women in industrialized societies in the past. It is an experience, moreover, which has seen considerable changes in the social organization of obstetric care and support within a society. As we examine contemporary pregnancy and studies in some of the areas highlighted above we will argue that a full understanding of this change can only occur if we examine the interaction between social, psychological and biological factors in the process and experience of pregnancy.

Medicalization of pregnancy

The medicalization of pregnancy is characterized by changing relationships of power between pregnant women and their professional carers during pregnancy and is marked by its potential for change. Medicalization has occurred as medical understanding of the biological process of pregnancy has increased along with its ability to intervene in the process. Widespread surveillance of pregnancy and childbirth now exists in industrialized societies. Nearly all women in such societies attend for prenatal care and are subject to medical monitoring and support throughout their pregnancy; the majority give birth in hospitals where obstetric technologies and medical interventions have increased massively over the last 30 years. The history of these changes, however, is a chequered one and highlights the social nature of science with inter-professional conflicts and the social and political nature of health care being as apparent as the claim of a neutral scientific approach to pregnancy (Stacey, 1988; Oakley, 1993). Sociologists, and feminists in particular, have been concerned to examine this feature of medical understanding of pregnancy, and how it has affected the social organization of obstetric care, its impact on women's experience of pregnancy and the varied ways in which women and health professionals have responded to the changes (Graham and Oakley, 1986; Oakley, 1984; Oakley, 1993; McIntosh, 1989; Romalis, 1985).

The medical model of pregnancy tends to claim a neutral scientific approach. It views pregnancy and childbirth as inherently problematic, requiring medical intervention and control in order to be accomplished successfully. Oakley (1993) argues that it is only by this transformation of the 'normal' to the 'potentially abnormal' that doctors have legitimized obstetrics as a medical speciality. As obstetrics and the medical model have gained credibility, alternative views of pregnancy as a natural event have declined, as has women's control over pregnancy. The dominance of the medical model leads to a dominant mechanical image of pregnant women and an assessment of pregnancy outcomes largely in terms of infant or maternal mortality rather than in terms of satisfaction or measures of positive health.

A number of writers have shown that women's assessment of pregnancy and childbirth often conflict with this 'neutral' view of doctors. Using evidence from samples of mothers in York and London, Graham and Oakley (1986) showed that the frames of reference of obstetricians and of women differed both as to the nature of childbearing and its context. Their studies showed that obstetricians use a relatively limited view of 'woman as patient' throughout pregnancy whereas women tended to view pregnancy not as an isolated episode but as integral with the rest of their lives. Such differences were seen by the mothers to lead to conflict at times. Oakley points out that the typical encounter between pregnant women and their obstetricians generally left the consultant in charge and prevented many women from voicing their questions and anxieties (Oakley, 1993).

A factor seen as important in restricting the possibility of women articulating their criticism is that of the power and authority of obstetricians. Indeed Romalis (1985) suggests that there is little evidence of disagreement with the medical model for the later stages of pregnancy – many women have come to accept that birth should be in a hospital and that technology is desirable. McIntosh (1989) sees this as determined more by class than simply gender and professionalization. Whereas studies of middle-class women tended to find marked dissatisfaction with the medicalized aspects of pregnancy and birth, e.g. Oakley (1990), McIntosh's study of 68 working-class pregnant women in Scotland in 1982 found that the great majority accepted the medicalization of birth and tended to accept the system they were given on the basis that the prevailing system must be the best. Nevertheless the 1980s saw considerable change in women's acceptance of the medicalization of childbirth and the medical profession has had to respond to a strong consumer movement in maternity care, and listen to the demands of women for greater participation in the management of pregnancy (Oakley, 1993).

The subsequent changes have largely been in relation to the care of women during the early and middle stages of pregnancy rather than affecting childbirth and technological surveillance at that stage. One example of an attempt to give some power back to women in the management of pregnancy and to increase their satisfaction has been in the amount of information that they are given during early visits to hospital. Lovell and colleagues (1986) report on such an innovation at St Thomas's hospital in London where half of a group of 246 mothers were given responsibility for looking after their maternity case notes between clinics, the rest simply holding less informative maternity 'co-operation' cards. Having the notes did appear to increase information sharing between mother and hospital staff, and maternal participation in decision-making. There was also some evidence that husbands and partners who read the notes, were better at providing companionship during labour and were more positive about involvement with the baby following birth. Similar benefits for mothers have been found in studies by Flint and Poulengeris and by Oakley. Flint and Poulengeris (1987) studied the effectiveness of providing continuous personal support from a midwife throughout pregnancy, Oakley (1992) studied the effectiveness of providing social support to women at risk of delivering low weight babies. In both studies women who received social support and increased information from midwives felt more in control during labour after this support, had slightly bigger babies and experienced better psychological health post partum.

The goal of maintaining a high level of information for mothers may be something that many women from all classes want and from which they and their babies would benefit. Unfortunately, despite the growth in the consumer move-ment in medical care, extending such care through pregnancy and especially extending it to choices about childbirth may prove to be more difficult. The St Thomas' innovation was successful because it had considerable support from the consultant and medical staff. Where such support is lacking the effects might not be so positive. Obstetrician's status depends on far more than patient satisfaction and as there are continual pressures on them to measure up in other scales, there may be little incentive for change. Not only does pregnancy occur within a social context, so also does medical care and the politics and social divisions of maternal medical care are highly significant in its development (Witz, 1990).

Psychological aspects of pregnancy

As pregnancy and childbirth have become safer and less frequent events, so the emphasis in research has shifted from factors affecting survival to those concerned with the psychosocial aspects of the experience. Pregnancy has been variously viewed by psychologists as a time of crisis brought about by emotional, psychological and social stress and reflecting the identity crisis of becoming a mother (Bibring, 1959); a period of fulfilment and calm in which a woman's deepest yearnings for motherhood and female achievement are met (Deutsch, 1947) or as a transitional phase in life akin to adolescence which marks the physical, social and psychological transition from non-motherhood to motherhood (Breen, 1975; Wolkind and Zajicek, 1981). Empirical findings drawn from studies using a range of methodologies including surveys, interviews, the use of standardized questionnaires and psychiatric interview, suggest that pregnancy is a time of mixed emotions. For example Green, 1990, who sampled a large, broadly representative group of pregnant English women, found that early in pregnancy 74% felt happy and 46% felt anxious. Similarly, Elliot and colleagues (1983) and Condon (1987) found a range of reactions to pregnancy, varying from increased emotional well-being to reports of depression and anxiety which were of a severity commensurate with psychiatric disorder. Longitudinal studies find that psychological reactions to pregnancy vary over its course (Wolkind and Zajicek, 1981).

As is usual in psychology, the focus of investigation has been on negative aspects of pregnancy – on 'problems' – rather than on positive aspects. Thus we know less about the range and intensity of happiness, joy, delight, energy and enthusiasm in pregnancy than we know about depression, anxiety, stress, tiredness and dread.

Unplanned pregnancy

Within this context, one particular focus of study has concerned the woman's feelings about being pregnant, the supposition being that an unwanted pregnancy would give rise to a host of negative psychological symptoms during pregnancy and birth and result in poor adjustment to motherhood. While the incidence of unwanted pregnancy has been reduced in many countries by the availability of effective contraception, rates of unplanned pregnancy remain high amongst some groups in certain societies. In the USA, for example, conception rates amongst the under twenties have seen a slow but steady increase between the 1970s and the 1990s. This increase does not necessarily mean an increase in unplanned pregnancies but the difference between the numbers becoming pregnant and the numbers giving birth in this age group suggest a large number of unplanned and unwanted events. In 1983 one teenage woman in ten was estimated to become pregnant, although only one in twenty gave birth (Pittman, 1986). At the same time in England and Wales only one teenage woman in eighteen was estimated to become pregnant; one in twenty-seven went on to give birth (OPCS, 1985). In older mothers, unplanned pregnancies are also common but often these births are highly desired.

Unplanned pregnancy should not therefore be equated with unwanted pregnancy, making the examination of the relationship between the desirability of pregnancy and psychological symptomatology difficult. A classic longitudinal study of pregnancy reinforces this point. Wolkind and Zajicek (1981) interviewed 247 primiparous (giving birth to their first baby) women from the East End of London, age 16 years and over about their attitudes to being pregnant, using standardized interview techniques. Thirty-one percent of the pregnancies were unplanned but only 10% of these women felt negative about their pregnancy both initially and at seven months. Wolkind and Zajicek found that their subjects' attitudes to being pregnant often changed as the pregnancy progressed. Thus women who initially had an unplanned and unwanted pregnancy were frequently reconciled to being pregnant by the time of the seven-month interview to the extent that the pregnancy was clearly welcomed and the birth eagerly anticipated. In contrast some women who felt very positively when they first found out they were pregnant, reported substantial negative feelings and attitudes to pregnancy in the later interview.

Some theorists, influenced by psychosomatic models of illness have further suggested that the psychological conflicts caused by an unwanted pregnancy could be manifest in physical symptoms of pregnancy and birth such as severe and long lasting morning sickness (hyperaemis gravis) or hypertension, however Wolkind and Zajicek (1981) found little empirical support for this hypothesis. Some indication of the complex relationship between physical, psychological and social adjustment to pregnancy can be gained from looking at their data on nausea and vomiting in pregnancy. Nausea and vomiting at any point in pregnancy was unrelated to any psychological rejection of the fetus. In early pregnancy it was unrelated to marital status, psychological dysfunction or psychiatric disorder, but nausea which continued throughout the pregnancy was more likely to be associated with psychiatric disorder if the woman was unmarried or if the woman was unsupported by her partner and/or family (Wolkind and Zajicek, 1981). Similar social influences relating to age and marital status have been found associated with distress in pregnancy (Gotlib, Whiffen, Mount et al., 1989; Lederman, 1984). Such bio-psycho-social analysis contributes to our understanding of how the dynamics of pregnancy change over its course.

Prenatal depression

A current topic of interest encompassed by the focus on negative aspects of pregnancy concerns the relationship between pre-pregnancy, prenatal and postnatal affective disorder, especially that involving depression. Research suggests that what was once regarded as an exclusively postnatal phenomenon – that of so-called postnatal depression – may have prenatal precursors, in that it is more likely to occur in women who report high levels of anxiety and depression in pregnancy (e.g. Watson, Elliot, Rugg and Brough, 1984; Sharp, 1989). Furthermore, a proportion of such women have a long-standing history of affective disorder or other indications of psychiatric morbidity not associated with reproduction (Sharp, 1989; Wolkind and Zajicek, 1981). Thus research in this area indicates that affective disturbance in pregnancy and in the postnatal period may in some women reflect the exacerbation of an underlying psychological vulnerability. This exacerbation may be due to hormonal factors or to the effects of the physical and psychological stresses inherent in reproduction (see below).

Compliance with prenatal health guidelines

Psychological research has not merely concerned itself with understanding the negative aspects of pregnancy. A major thrust of recent research has been directed towards the relief of distress or the alleviation of problems. While the relief of distress is centred on the woman's own experience and is discussed in the section on stress in pregnancy, the 'problems' which have been addressed have often been defined by the health care system or by society. For example 'non-compliance' with prenatal health care guidelines on diet and on restrictions in alcohol, tobacco and other drug use concerns health practitioners and policy makers (e.g. National Institute of Child Health and Human Development, 1990) but may not concern the woman herself who may gain short-term benefits from smoking, drinking or eating cream cakes.

Demographic factors which might predict non-compliance have been investigated but no clear relationship between them has been found. Psychological factors including health beliefs and health locus of control also show no consistent relationship with prenatal behaviour patterns (Rutter and Quine, 1990; Tinsley and Holtgrave, 1989). However studies which examine women's beliefs about control over the health of the fetus or over pregnancy and birth outcomes, have demonstrated significant relationships with prenatal behaviours involving smoking and caffeine intake (Labs and Wurtele, 1986) and compliance with a prenatal care regime related to risky behaviour in pregnancy including alcohol and drug use (Tinsley, Turpin, Owens and Boyum, 1993). The latter study found that women who perceived that they had control over pregnancy and birth outcomes were more 'compliant' and had better pregnancy outcome. However, few direct relationships were found between health beliefs, specific prenatal behaviour patterns and pregnancy outcome, and the amount of variance accounted for was small. Thus the multiple factors which affect the processes by which pregnancy beliefs influence prenatal behaviour remain to be elucidated. Sociodemographic factors are likely to be involved as health attitudes are commonly found to vary across class, ethnic and cultural groups (Tinsley, Turpin, Owens and Boyum, 1993). Furthermore there is some suggestion that obstetric factors such as previous reproductive loss may relate to health beliefs about the fetus (Bielawaska-Batorowicz, 1993).

Stress in pregnancy

There are a wide range of potential stressors that attach to pregnancy. Although its physical risks have been considerably reduced, they have not been eliminated. Furthermore, screening for fetal abnormality has highlighted risks which had previously been hidden or were at least less apparent to the pregnant woman. Considerable adaptation to physical and psychosocial changes during pregnancy is also required.

Stress in pregnancy, as outwith pregnancy manifests itself in psychological symptoms psychologically. The principal symptoms are anxiety, depression and irritability which have been found in pregnant women experiencing stressful life events and in those whose pregnancies are threatened with miscarriage, stillbirth or fetal abnormality (Condon, 1987; Fearn, Hibbard, Laurence, et al., 1982). Screening procedures which indicate possible abnormality are associated with intense anxiety (Fearn, Hibbard, Laurence, et al., 1982). High levels of anxiety in pregnancy are also related to the previous experience of miscarriage, stillbirth, neonatal death, handicap or prematurity (Mandell and Wolff, 1975; Helper, Cohen, Beitenman and Eaton, 1968; van den Akker, Sweeny and Rosenblatt, 1990). The stressful effects of pregnancy have also been highlighted in men whose partners are pregnant, with raised levels of anxiety, irritability and depression being found in fathers-to-be (Condon, 1987), and men expressing fears about the possible dangers which face their partners and worries about the changes that pregnancy and birth will bring for their relationship (Lewis, 1986).

Physically, the reactions to stress have effects not only on the mother but also potentially on the fetus as stress hormones, particularly the catecholamines, can affect uterine blood supply and muscle contractibility and pass through the placental barrier to affect the fetus (Lederman, Lederman, Work and McCann, 1978). As association between severe stress in pregnancy, resulting from such stressful life events as serious illness in a close family member, and low birth weight and premature delivery has been partially attributed to these physical effects of stress (Newton and Hunt, 1984; Newton, 1988). Stress in pregnancy may also have indirect, harmful consequences for mother and fetus since Newton and Hunt's study showed that smoking and poor clinic attendance were more likely in mothers suffering severe stress, and were associated with low birth weight. More recent studies have not found a relationship between the number of life events per se and pregnancy outcome but between the perceived stress-fullness of these events and low birth weight and premature delivery (Lobel, Dunkell-Schetter and Scrimshaw, 1992). This suggests that stress in pregnancy is best viewed within the cognitive appraisal framework; i.e. as resulting from the individual's appraisal of stress, rather than as an inevitable consequence of encountering a stressful event or experience (Lazarus and Folkman, 1984). The effects of coping resources in mediating the appraisal of stress are central to this framework and are discussed below.

Current psychophysiological models of stress (e.g. Frankenhauser, 1983) which take as a starting point the appraisal process and link this to both physiological and psychological outcomes, can thus be applied to pregnancy (see Figure 4.1). These demonstrate clearly the benefits of considering pregnancy from a biopsychological perspective. Such a model however lacks a social framework. The experience of pregnancy takes place in an intimate social context – that of the family – and in the context of the wider society.

The family

Pregnancy automatically occurs in a family setting, whether defined legally, socially or biologically (Niven, 1992). The reactions of family members to the women's pregnancy, be they lovers, partners, children, parents or siblings can effect her experience. This effect can be set within the model of stress in

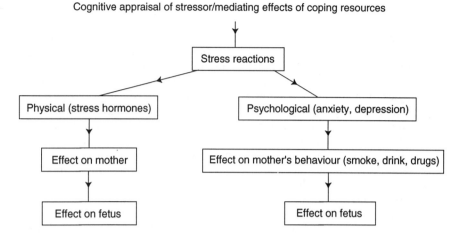

Figure 4.1 A psychophysiological model of stress in pregnancy.

pregnancy laid out in Figure 4.1. Poor relationships within a family can be a potent source of stress. For instance marital breakdown or rejection of the pregnancy by a male partner has been linked with poor maternal adjustment to pregnancy and prenatal depression; so has perceived lack of support from family, most notably the father-to-be (Helper, Cohen, Beitenman and Eaton, 1968; Scott-Heyes, 1984; Collins, Dunkell-Schetter, Lobel and Scrimshaw, 1993). But the family can also provide one of the major sources of social support in pregnancy. Debate continues over the mechanisms of social support in general and of social support in pregnancy in particular (Carrol, Niven and Sheffield, 1993). Within the family, social support may be instrumental, involving the provision of goods or assistance with tasks or may be emotional, transmitting feelings of being loved and cared about and boosting self-esteem. These forms of social support may offset the negative effects of stress as well as possibly having direct effects on maternal and thus fetal well-being (Collins, Dunkell-Schetter, Lobel and Scrimshaw, 1993).

The resources a family can draw upon to provide instrumental support for a pregnant family member may be determined by broad social policies which act to either 'enrich' or deprive the family of material resources at this time. Instrumental support may also be provided directly by the state, for example through income supplementation or help with domestic and child rearing tasks. Studies which have examined the outcome of such provision have demonstrated beneficial effects as measured by the birth weight of babies born to mothers known to be at risk of having low birth weight babies (Kotelchuck, Schwartz, Anderka and Finison, 1984; Papiernik, Bouyer and Dreyfus, 1985). Health professionals, government agencies, etc., may also provide information for families during pregnancy which may enable them to access sources of instrumental support. Thus, when considering the resources which are available to the pregnant woman which may benefit her directly or buffer the stress she is experiencing, the broader social context needs to be taken into account.

Society

The wider societal context of pregnancy has been of central concern to sociologists who have a particular interest in the way that societal factors may affect the stresses of pregnancy and the resources available to pregnant women (Dally, 1982; Phoenix, Woollett and Lloyd, 1991; Oakley, 1993). Changing ideologies of motherhood, patterns of inequality, family structures, professional practices and state policies are all factors that affect the transformation in women's roles produced by motherhood and the additional emotional and economic costs that are incurred. The sources of support that a woman can turn to in order to cope with these costs are varied, and sociologists have been concerned to show how they are affected by the ideological framework and material resources available to household and kin members (Phoenix, Woollett and Lloyd, 1991).

One study which gives some indication of recent changes in the social context of pregnancy and possible sources of support during the last 40 years is that of Thompson (1989). Focusing solely on married women, the study compares the experience of 200 women in Aberdeen whose first pregnancy ended in birth in either 1951 or 1985. The study shows an increase in available resources, making possible choices in areas such as housing, diet and social activities. There was clearly an increase in the material support available for the pregnant women. The comparison showed that couples in 1985 were more mobile than 40 years earlier, were more likely to have stayed on at school, had fewer housing problems, were more likely to be two income households prior to parenthood and to have wives in professional, technical and clerical occupations (73% compared with 30% in 1951). Although there has been some concern about the decline of kin and the isolation of young parents since the 1950s (Wilmot and Young, 1957) the Aberdeen study showed that about half of the sample still saw their mothers or mothers-in-law daily or several times a week, thus suggesting that social support is still available for some women from their kin. A particularly noticeable change between the studies concerned the changing involvement of husbands in their wives' pregnancy. In the 1950s, for example, there was an acceptance of the separate roles of men and women and any suggestion that men attended the birth was considered indecent. In 1981 husbands were expected to take an active role in the support of their wives during pregnancy, were included in antenatal classes and generally volunteered to accompany their wives during labour.

The Aberdeen study is specifically focused on married women and vividly shows the effect of raised standards of living on pregnancy in marriage. However we have to remember that such a group is declining. Marriage rates in the UK have dropped dramatically in the last 20 years and in Aberdeen itself married women represented 85% of births in 1951, but only 60% by 1985. There is no doubt that family life has changed considerably in the UK over recent years. Cohabitation has now become relatively common – in 1971 only 4% of births were registered outside marriage by both parents, by 1989 this had increased to one in five (Central Statistical Office, 1991). In the UK cohabitation still tends to precede marriage but the Swedish experience is of considerable numbers remaining unmarried even with children, and we must ask whether the attractions of marriage as a source of emotional and material support during pregnancy and childrearing are wearing thin (McRae, 1993).

But it is not just marriage that has changed. Economic change has produced not only the families with raised standards of living in Aberdeen, it has also paradoxically, produced an increase in households living in poverty. For example declining sources of employment and government unwillingness to provide income maintenance for the young as a whole was characteristic of the UK in the 1980s and 1990s and the resulting loss of resources might be expected to produce particular difficulties for young mothers. Phoenix's study of 79 young mothers found that the ability of young fathers and the parents to financially support and cope with pregnancy was severely limited and was more-over, related to levels of education and income. But she also found that emotional and practical support was often available from parents and partners of teenage mothers (Phoenix, 1991). Together with the evident network of social relation-ships and perception of caring by the mothers it would appear, from this study at least, that pregnancy can still be a positive experience for the young. Nevertheless, despite the considerable amount of emotional and practical support for all her sample during pregnancy, Phoenix found that two-thirds of the young mothers were experiencing financial problems or expected to have money prob-lems once their child was born.

One result of such financial worries seems to be a greater propensity to an activity commonly held to be unwise in pregnancy – smoking. In Graham's study of low-income households (1987) 28% of mothers reported using smoking as a coping strategy. Other work has confirmed this pattern and its occurrence, despite the fact that the mothers are aware of its impact on their own and their child's health (Oakley, 1989). In both studies it was found that smoking was used to compensate for poor material conditions and for low levels of emotional and practical support where they existed. Lack of material resources is an increasingly common feature of the life of many women with children in the UK (Glendinning and Millar, 1985). Payne (1991) comments that in the UK the cuts in benefits available to all women during pregnancy have resulted in a substantial increase in the risk of poverty at a time when standards of living are crucial for the healthy outcome of pregnancy. There are two factors, however which hide the increased vulnerability to poverty that women experience as they make the transition to motherhood. These are the high rate of employment for married women prior to motherhood and the dependence of women on the income of male partners. Where employment rates are low, or where there is no male partner, then vulnerability to poverty is particularly high.

What this highlights is the role of the state in mediating the resources available to pregnant women. In the 1970s Britain saw a welcome extension of maternity leave entitlements and increased maternity benefits. Unfortunately during the 1980s and 1990s there has been a continual erosion of those rights and an increasing economic vulnerability for pregnant women (Brannen and Moss, 1988). Universal maternity grant has been replaced by discretionary means-tested benefits, and the additional cost of maternity clothes and baby equipment has become difficult to achieve on benefit levels (Oppenheim, 1990; Roll, 1986). The end result has been an increased reliance on household earnings for maternal well-being. In consequence the number of women working until the third trimester of their pregnancy has increased recently in the UK. The interval between births has also decreased, presumably reflecting families' attempts to maximize their earnings by compressing their productive years into as short a timeframe as possible (Central Statistical Office, 1991; Oakley, 1993).

A father's role in pregnancy is also affected by changes in welfare legislation and maternity rights. The British government for example, has consistently refused to legislate on paternity leave, and entitlements for fathers are much the lowest in Europe. It means that the ability of men to support their partners, both materially and psychologically, is constrained by the state as well as by private arrangements between male workers and their employers. Nevertheless men are now present at various points of pregnancy in ways that were unthinkable 30 years ago. In the Aberdeen study of married couples (Thompson, 1989) husbands were expected to take an active part in preparing for parenthood. In contrast to 1950s, fathers in the 1980s were included in antenatal classes and their presence in the labour ward was considered advisable. There is, however, more rather than less evidence of an increase in gendered divisions of labour accompanying the development of pregnancy (Morris, 1990).

Clearly then economic and social change and the level of stress which women may experience in pregnancy is mediated by family, employer and state structures of support. Since we have already argued that stress has important physical and psychological consequences for women in pregnancy, changes in the structuring of support represent an important area for research. Unfortunately there has been relatively little in the way of such direct research.

Summary

Consideration of pregnancy from a bio-psycho-social perspective focuses attention on their complex inter-relationships. While biomedical advances have been notable, the psychological consequences of these have not always been favourable. These advances have also increased the medicalization of pregnancy which has profoundly altered attitudes to pregnancy within our society.

Pregnancy is often a joyous time or is at least a predominantly positive experience. However psychological concerns have been directed more to the negative aspects of pregnancy. Stress in pregnancy has formed a central concept in the psychology of pregnancy, just as stress is central to health psychology as a whole. What this chapter shows is that the effects of stress in pregnancy are wide-ranging, affecting both fetus and mother-to-be, and are therefore best considered within a psychobiological framework. The task of alleviating stress in pregnancy, however, directs our attention to the interdependent roles of the family, society and the state in providing the necessary resources.

As the forms of families have changed, so the labour market and the state have become increasingly important structures affecting the material and personal resources available to pregnant women and their families. Present moves away from many of the central tenets of welfare state; plus a growing dependence of households on women's earned income have meant that some groups of women are likely to experience more rather than less stress over the next few years.

The potential for changes in medical practice, for state legislation and welfare and for employment practices to alleviate stress during pregnancy needs to be considered if the experiences of pregnancy and its outcomes are to keep pace with biological improvements.

Applications

1. Many pregnancies are happy and healthy experiences, but it is necessary to recognize that stress can have a considerable effect on the experience and outcome of pregnancy.

2. The use and development of 'family support' strategies by community health professionals is recommended rather than strategies focused solely on the health of the fetus.

3. The use and development of 'woman friendly' obstetric practices is important, including measures that allow women some control in the management of their pregnancy.

4. The development of employment practices and state welfare that ensures adequate material resources during pregnancy is crucial along with sufficient incentives for partners to provide active support during pregnancy.

Further reading

Oakley, A. (1993). *Essays on Women, Medicine and Health.* Edinburgh: Edinburgh University Press.
Payne, S. (1991). *Women, Health and Poverty, an Introduction.* Hemel Hempstead: Wheatsheaf.
Phoenix, A., Woollett, A. and Lloyd, E. (1991). *Motherhood: meanings, practices and ideologies.* London: Sage.

References

Bibring, G. L. (1959). Some considerations of the psychological processes in pregnancy. *Psychoanalytic Study of the Child*, **14**, 113–21.
Bielawaska-Batorowicz, E. (1993). The effect of previous obstetric history on women's scores on the Fetal Health Locus of Control Scale. *Journal of Reproductive and Infant Psychology*, **11**, 103–7.
Brannen, J. and Moss, P. (1988). *New mothers at work.* London: Unwin Hyman.
Breen, D. (1975). *The Birth of a First Child.* London: Tavistock Publications.
Carrol, D., Niven, C. and Sheffield, D. (1993). Gender, health and social circumstances. In *The Health Psychology of Women* (C. A. Niven and D. Carroll, eds). Switzerland: Harwood Academic Publishers.
Central Statistical Office (1991). *Social Trends*, **21**, London: HMSO.
Collins, N., Dunkell-Schetter, C., Lobel, M. and Scrimshaw, S. (1993). Social Support in pregnancy: Psychological correlates of birth outcomes and postpartum depression. *Journal of Personality and Social Psychology*, **65**, 1243–58.
Condon, J. T. (1987). Psychological and physical symptoms during pregnancy: A comparison of male and female expectant parents. *Journal of Reproductive and Infant Psychology*, **5**, 207–13.

Currer, C. (1986). Health concepts and illness behaviour: the care of Pathan mothers in Britain. Unpublished PhD thesis. University of Warwick.

Dally, A. (1982). *Inventing Motherhood*. London: Hutchison.

Deutsch, H. (1947). *The Psychology of Women*. New York: Grune and Stratton.

Elliot, S. A., Rugg, A. J., Watson, J. P. and Brough, D. I. (1983). Mood changes during pregnancy and after the birth of a child. *British Journal of Clinical Psychology*, **22**, 295–308.

Fearn, J., Hibbard, B. M., Laurence, K. M., Roberts, A. and Robinson, J. D. (1982). Screening for neural tube defects and maternal anxiety. *British Journal of Obstetrics and Gynaecology*, **89**, 218–21.

Flint, C. and Poulengeris, P. (1987). *The 'Know your midwife scheme'*. London: report published by authors.

Frankenhauser, M. (1983). The sympathetic-adrenal and pituitary-adrenal response to challenge: comparison between the sexes. In *Bio-Behavioral Bases of Coronary Heart Disease* (T. M. Dembrowsky, T. Schmidt and G. Blumchen, eds). Basel: Carger.

Glendinning, M. and Millar, N. (1985). *Women and Poverty in Britain*. Sussex: Wheatsheaf.

Gotlib, I. H., Whiffen, V. E., Mount, T. H., Milne, K. and Cordy, N. I. (1989). Prevalence rates and demographic characteristics associated with depression in pregnancy and the postpartum. *Journal of Consulting and Clinical Psychology*, **57**, 269–74.

Graham, H. (1987). Women's smoking and family health. *Social Science and Medicine*, **25**, 45–56.

Graham, H. and Oakley, A. (1986). Competing ideologies of reproduction: medical and maternal perspectives on pregnancy. In *Concepts of Health, Illness and Disease* (C. Currer, and M. Stacey, eds). Oxford: Berg.

Green, J. M. (1990). Is the baby alright and other worries. Paper presented at the 10th Anniversary Conference of the Society for Reproductive and Infant Psychology, Cambridge, England.

Halinka Maloe, L. (1994). National policy, social conditions and the etiology of maternal mortality. *Epidemiology*, **5**, 481–3.

Helper, M. M., Cohen, R. L., Beitenman, E. T. and Eaton, L. F. (1968). Life events and acceptance of pregnancy. *Journal of Psychosomatic Research*, **12**, 183–8.

Kotelchuck, M., Schwartz, J., Anderka, M. and Finison, K. (1984). WIC participation and pregnancy outcomes. *American Journals of Public Health*, **74**, 1086–92.

Labs, S. M., Wurtele, S. K. (1986). Fetal Health Locus of Control Scale: development and validation. *Journal of Consulting and Clinical Psychology*, **54**, 814–19.

Lazarus, R. and Folkman, S. (1984). *Stress, Appraisal and Coping*. New York: Springer.

Lederman, R. P. (1984). Anxiety and conflict in pregnancy: relationship to maternal health status. *Annual Review of Nursing Research*, **2**, 27–61.

Lederman, R. P., Lederman, E., Work, B. A. and McCann, D. S. (1978). The relationship of maternal anxiety, plasma catecholamines and plasma cortisol to progress in labour. *American Journal of Obstetrics and Gynaecology*, **132**, 495–500.

Lewis, C. (1986). *Becoming a Father*. Milton Keynes: Open University Press.

Lewis, J. (1980). *The Politics of Motherhood, Child and Maternal Welfare in England 1900–3*. Montreal: McGill-Queens University Press.

Llewelyn Davies, M. (ed.) (1978). *Maternity: Letters from working women*. London: Virago.

Lobel, M., Dunkell-Schetter, N. and Scrimshaw, B. (1992). Prenatal maternal stress and prematurity: prospective study of socio-economically disadvantaged women. *Health Psychology*, **11**, 32–40.

Loudon, I. (1992a). *Death in Childbirth. An international study of maternal care and maternal mortality, 1800–1950*. Oxford: Oxford University Press.

Loudon, I. (1992b). The transformation of maternal mortality. *British Medical Journal*, **305**, 1557–60.

Lovell, A., Zander, L. and Chamberlain, G. (1986). *St Thomas Maternity Case Notes Study: Why not give mothers their own case notes*. London: Cicely Northcote Trust.

Mandell, F. and Wolff, L. (1975). Sudden infant death syndrome and subsequent pregnancy. *Pediatrics*, **56**, 774–6.

McIntosh, J. (1989). Models of childbirth and social class: a study of 80 working class primigravidae. In *Midwives, Research and Childbirth* (S. Robinson and A. Thompson, eds). London: Chapman and Hall.

McRae, S. (1993). *Cohabiting Mothers: Changing marriage and motherhood?* London: PSI.

Morris, L. (1990). *The Workings of the Household.* Cambridge: Polity Press.

Morse, J. M. (1989). Cultural variation in behavioural response to parturition: Childbirth in Fiji. *Medical Anthropology,* **12,** 35–54.

Newton, R. W. (1988). Psychosocial aspects of pregnancy: the scope for intervention. *Journal of Reproductive and Infant Psychology,* **6,** 23–39.

Newton, R. W. and Hunt, L. P. (1984). Psychosocial stress in pregnancy and its relation to low birth weight. *British Medical Journal,* **288,** 1191–4.

National Institute of Child Health and Human Development (1990). *Care for our future: the content of prenatal care.* A report of the Public Health Service expert panel on the context of prenatal care. Bethesda, MD: National Institutes of Health.

Ni, H. and Rossignol, A. M. (1994). Maternal deaths among women with pregnancies outside of family planning in Sichuan, China. *Epidemiology,* **5,** 490–4.

Niven, C. (1992). *Psychological Care for Families: Before, During and After Birth.* Oxford: Butterworth-Heinemann.

Oakley, A. (1984). *The Captured Womb: a History of the Medical Care of Pregnant Women.* Oxford: Blackwell.

Oakley, A. (1989). Smoking in pregnancy: smokescreen or risk factor? Toward a materialist analysis. *Sociology of Health and Illness,* **11,** 311–32.

Oakley, A. (1990). *Women Confined: towards a sociology of childbirth.* Oxford: M. Robertson.

Oakley, A. (1992). *Social Support and Motherhood: the natural history of a research project.* Oxford: Basil Blackwell.

Oakley, A. (1993). *Essays on Women, Medicine and Health.* Edinburgh: Edinburgh University Press.

OPCS (1985). Trends in conceptions in England and Wales during 1983, *OPCS Monitor.* Reference FM1 86/2.

Oppenheim, C. (1990). *Poverty: the Facts.* London: Child Poverty Action Group.

Papiernik, E., Bouyer, J. and Drefus, J. (1985). Risk factors for pre-term births and results of a prevention policy. In *Preterm labor and its consequences* (R. W. Beard and F. Sharp, eds). Proceedings of 13th study group, Royal College of Obstetricians and Gynaecologists. Manchester: R. Bates.

Payne, S. (1991). *Women, Health and Poverty, an Introduction.* Hemel Hempstead: Wheatsheaf.

Phoenix, A. (1991). *Young Mothers.* Oxford: Polity Press.

Phoenix, A., Woollett, A. and Lloyd, E. (1991). *Motherhood: meanings, practices and ideologies.* London: Sage.

Pittman, K. (1986). *Adolescent Pregnancy, whose problem is it?* Washington: Children's Defense Fund's Adolescent Pregnancy Clearing House.

Roll, J. (1986). *Dear Mother? Maternity Payments Reform.* London: Family Policy Studies Centre.

Romalis, R. (1985). Struggle between providers and recipients: the case of birth practices. In *Women, Health and Healing* (E. Lewin and V. Olese, eds). London: Tavistock.

Rutter, D. R. and Quine, L. (1990). Inequalities in pregnancy outcome: a review of psycho social and behavioural mediators. *Social Science and Medicine,* **30,** 553–68.

Scott-Heyes, G. (1984). Childbearing as a mutual experience. Unpublished D. Phil thesis. New University of Ulster.

Sharp, D. J. (1989). Emotional disorders during pregnancy and the puerperium – a longitudinal prospective study in Primary Care. *Marce Society Bulletin*: Spring issue.

Stacey, M. (1988). *The Sociology of Health and Healing.* London: Hyman.

Thompson, A. (1989). *Having a first baby: experiences in 1951 and 1985 compared: two social, obstetric and dietary studies of married primagravidae in Aberdeen.* Aberdeen: Aberdeen University Press.

Tinsley, B. and Holtgrave, D. R. (1989). Maternal health locus of control beliefs, utilisation of child preventative health services and infant health. *Journal of Developmental and Behavioral Pediatrics,* **10,** 236–41.

Tinsley, B., Trupin, S., Owens, M. and Boyum, L. (1993). The significance of women's pregnancy-related locus of control beliefs for adherence to recommended prenatal health regimens and pregnancy outcomes. *Journal of Reproductive and Infant Psychology,* **11,** 97–102.

Van den Akker, O., Sweeny, V. and Rosenblatt, D. (1990). Psychological factors associated with pregnancy and the postnatal period in women at risk for preterm labour/delivery. Poster presented at the 10th Anniversary Conference of the Society for Reproductive and Infant Psychology. Cambridge, England.

Watson, J. P., Elliot, S. A., Rugg, A. H. and Brough, D. I. (1984). Psychiatric disorder in pregnancy and the first postnatal year. *British Journal of Psychiatry*, **144**, 453–62.

Wilmot, P. and Young, M. (1957). *Family and Kinship in East London.* London: Routledge and Kegan Paul.

Witz, A. (1990). *Professions and Patriarchy.* London: Routledge.

Wolkind, S. and Zajicek, E. (1981). *Pregnancy: A Psychological and Social Study.* London: Academic Press.

5

The fetus during pregnancy

Peter Hepper

This chapter complements Chapter 4 in examining pregnancy from the perspective of the fetus, rather than the mother. Until very recently, little was known about the behaviour and responses of the fetus, except as reflected in the mother's reports of the activity she could feel. The advent of ultrasound scanning has revolutionized this area of study and in this chapter Peter Hepper presents us with a fascinating view of pregnancy from the perspective of the fetus. Increased knowledge about fetal abilities not only pushes the frontiers of developmental psychology back in time, with the familiar debates about neonate abilities reappearing in a new 'prenatal' guise, but also raises many controversial moral and ethical issues. As such, this chapter casts new light on aspects of prenatal intervention and care and on prematurity.

Introduction

The prenatal period marks the most rapid time of development of our lives. Whilst the physical development of the fetus has been extensively documented, its behavioural and psychological development has, by comparison, received very little scientific study. It is the intention of the following chapter to review these aspects of fetal development.

Views on the abilities of the fetus have varied between two extremes. At one extreme the fetus has been viewed as a passive entity, developing only physically, in an environment devoid of stimulation or unresponsive to any stimulation that may be present. At the other extreme the fetus is seen as a fully sentient, conscious individual possessed of all the abilities of the adult. Only recently has scientific attention turned to study the behavioural development of the fetus, to accurately describe the fetus's abilities.

The renewed interest in the development of the fetus may be attributed, largely, to two factors: advances in the study of the newborn infant and improved methods of observing the fetus.

For many years the newborn was considered immature and incapable of most perceptual and learning abilities. Part of the reason for this view was the inappropriate methodology adopted in studying the newborn. Researchers initially applied techniques used with adults to explore their abilities but the immature response system of the newborn was unable to cope with the demands of the task, leading researchers to conclude that newborns possessed few abilities. However as experimental techniques become more sophisticated and matched to the response capabilities of the newborn, the abilities of the newborn were revealed to be more advanced than previously thought. Today newborns are known to have well-developed sensory systems in all modalities; visual, auditory, cutaneous, olfactory and gustatory, and have been demonstrated to possess a wide variety of learning abilities; exposure/familiarity, instrumental, classical and imitation (Diamond, 1990). Questions were thus raised regarding the ontogenesis of these abilities. It was possible, although unlikely, that they arose *de novo* at the moment of birth. More likely was the fact that these abilities arose some time during the prenatal period, commencing their development then, with birth merely marking a transition from their exhibition *in utero* to their exhibition *ex utero*. Researchers thus turned their attention to the prenatal period to study the ontogenesis of fetal behavioural and psychological abilities.

A second important reason behind the resurgence of interest in the prenatal period was the development of ultrasound technology enabling the non-invasive visualization of the fetus in real time (Hepper, 1990). Prior to this development, observation of the fetus relied on devices such as: stethoscopes, to 'hear' the fetus; strain gauges, to record fetal movements via their effect on the maternal abdomen, and; the oldest method, maternal perception of fetal movement. Although these methods provided some indication of fetal activities, ultrasound opened a completely new window of observation by providing accurate pictures of the fetus (Dewbury, Meire and Cosgrove, 1993). The resolution of the current generation of ultrasound machine is such that it is possible to observe the opening and closing of the pupil of the fetus's eye. This has enabled the behaviour of the fetus to be studied in great detail.

Whilst these advances have lead to increased study of the human fetus over the past 10–15 years, interest in the psychological development of the fetus has been present for many centuries (Hepper, 1992a). Aristotle in *De Generatione Animalium* argued that the fetus could experience its environment and Súsruta, the Indian scientist writing in the 6th century BC, proposed that the fetus was able to sense its environment at 12 weeks of gestational age (GA). Both Empedocles, 450 BC, and Caraka, 1000 BC, thought the fetus could be affected by the mental state of the mother. There are numerous references in the Bible to prenatal experiences influencing development (e.g. Genesis 31: 30–43) and over 1000 years ago the Chinese established 'prenatal clinics' to ensure the psychological health of the fetus (Ellis, 1940).

The study of fetal behaviour

The earliest stages of development are still shrouded in mystery. A greater understanding of the behaviour of the fetus is important for progress in a number of scientific and clinical lines of enquiry.

First, and obviously, little is known about the prenatal behavioural development of the fetus and hence there is the need for more information on all aspects of prenatal behavioural ontogenesis, i.e. the origin and development of an individual's behaviour. The behaviour of the fetus needs to be described to enable the ontogenetic processes underlying fetal development to be elucidated and the antecedents of postnatal behaviour to be identified.

Second, the behaviour of the individual reflects its underlying neural structure (e.g. Hepper, 1992a; Nijhuis, 1986). Thus inferences can be made regarding the individual's prenatal neural development from observation of its behaviour providing evidence of the relationship, and interaction, between neural structure and function.

Third, advances in medical technology have greatly reduced the mortality and morbidity of premature infants. Individuals born at 24 weeks' GA now stand a good chance of survival. However future improvements in the care of these infants requires a greater understanding of their behaviour and that of the fetus and its environment to promote appropriate regimes which foster normal development.

Finally, a greater understanding of fetal behaviour may enable the health of the fetus to be more accurately assessed (Hepper, 1990). As the behaviour of the fetus directly reflects the functioning of its nervous system, observation of fetal behaviour may enable the integrity of the nervous system to be assessed and hence the well-being of the fetus to be evaluated.

Fetal behavioural development

Motor development

Early studies examining human fetal movements were performed on aborted fetuses (Minkowski, 1928) where the first movements were seen at 12 weeks' GA. This corresponds to the time the first fetal movements were 'heard' using a stethoscope (Preyer, 1885). Later studies (Hooker, 1952; Humphrey, 1978) reported movements beginning at around 7 weeks' GA. Although these observations were performed on aborted, and thus essentially dying, fetuses they demonstrated that the first movements of the fetus occurred very early during gestation.

The first study using ultrasound, performed by Reinold (1971), observed fetal movements at 8 weeks' GA. Since this study others have confirmed that the first fetal movements are seen at 7–8 weeks' GA. These have been described as 'rippling' movements (van Dongen and Goudie, 1980), 'vermicular' movements (Ianniruberto and Tajani, 1981), a 'twitch' (Birnholz, Stevens and Faria, 1978), 'just discernible' movements (de Vries, Visser and Prechtl, 1982, 1985). Although given different descriptors by their various authors the appearance of these movements on ultrasound is more uniform where they appear as slow movements, originating in the back or spinal column, causing it to flex or extend, and possibly resulting in passive movements of the arms and legs.

De Vries, Visser and Prechtl (1982, 1985) described the development of individual movements over the first half of pregnancy. From the first movements at 7–8 weeks' GA, the next few weeks see the emergence of over 20 different movements. The first appearance of these movements is documented in Table 5.1. Each particular motor behaviour has its own developmental time-course. Thus, for example, sucking increases in frequency over the first half of pregnancy whilst startles decline in frequency after 8/9 weeks' GA. By 20 weeks' GA the fetus exhibits the same basic motor patterns as found in term and pre-term infants. As gestation proceeds these movements become increasingly more complex and structured, and individual movements become more refined and co-ordinated in their occurrence. There is no difference between the movements of males and females although individuals of both sexes exhibit large inter-individual differences (de Vries, Visser and Prechtl, 1988).

Two specific types of movements, eye movements and breathing movements, have attracted attention.

At 16 weeks' GA the first fetal eye movements can be observed (Birnholz, 1981) initially occurring as slow eye movements. But at 23 weeks' GA rapid eye movements may be observed (Horimoto, Hepper, Shahidullah and Koyanagi, 1993).

Table 5.1

Behaviour	Gestational Age (wks)
Just discernible movement	7
Startle	8
General movement	8
Hiccup	9
Isolated arm movement	9
Isolated leg movement	9
Isolated head movement	9
Isolated head rotation	9–10
Isolated head anteflexion	10
Fetal breathing movements	10
Arm twitch	10
Leg twitch	10
Hand-face contact	10
Stretch	10
Rotation of fetus	10
Jaw movement	10–11
Yawn	11
Finger movement	12
Sucking and swallowing	12
Clonic movement arm or leg	13
Rooting	14
Eye movements	16

The gestational age at which behaviours are first observed in the fetus (adapted from Birnholz 1981; de Vries et al. 1982, 1985).

Movements described as fetal breathing movements are somewhat paradoxical as there is no air in the fetus's fluid-filled uterine environment for it to breathe. However the movements observed, motions of the diaphragm and rib cage, would result in breathing after birth and hence are termed fetal breathing movements. At 9 weeks' GA the first breathing movements are observed and are regular in nature (de Vries, Visser and Prechtl, 1985). Irregular breathing movements appear at 12 weeks' GA (de Vries, Visser and Prechtl, 1985). By 30 weeks' GA fetal breathing movements are episodic in nature and occur around 30% of the time (Patrick, Campbell, Carmichael et al., 1980).

During the first trimester of pregnancy movements are randomly distributed. However, during the second trimester rest–activity cycles are observed, with increasing periods of time where no activity occurs being observed with advancing gestation (Pillai, James and Parker, 1992).

During the last 3–4 weeks of pregnancy behavioural states have been observed in the fetus (Nijhuis, Prechtl, Martin and Bots, 1982). Four behavioural states (numbered 1F–4F, F representing fetal) have been identified, following observations of behavioural states in newborns (Prechtl, 1974). Three 'independent' variables are used to define a behavioural state, heart rate, eye movements and body movements (Nijhuis, Prechtl, Martin and Bots, 1982). These variables were chosen from work which demonstrated they could be used to identify behavioural states in the newborn infant (Prechtl and Beintema, 1964). The four states are:

- **State 1F**: Quiescence, occasional startles; no eye movements; stable fetal heart rate (pattern A).

- **State 2F**: Frequent and periodic gross body movements; eye movements present; fetal heart rate shows frequent accelerations in association with movement (pattern B).
- **State 3F**: No gross body movements; eye movements present; fetal heart rate (pattern C) shows no accelerations and has a wider oscillation bandwidth than State 1F (although some have questioned the existence of this particular state) (Pillai and James, 1990)).
- **State 4F**: Continual activity; eye movements present; fetal heart rate unstable and tachycardia present (pattern D).

The emergence of these stable patterns of behaviour has been argued to represent a greater degree of integration between the various centres of the central nervous system (Nijhuis, 1986).

Summary

The first fetal movements are observed very early during gestation and by mid-gestation a stable repertoire of individual movements is emitted by the fetus. During the second half of gestation, fetal behaviour becomes organized into rest–activity cycles, culminating in the exhibition of behavioural states in the final weeks of pregnancy. These movements are mediated by the spontaneous activity of the fetus's nervous system and the observed maturation of motor patterns corresponds to the maturation of the nervous system and higher neural centres exerting greater control over motor output.

Sensory development

The sensory abilities of the fetus must be considered with respect to two aspects. First, whether the fetus can respond to a particular stimulus, and second whether such stimulation would be present normally in the fetal environment.

Audition

The ease with which auditory stimuli may be presented to the fetus (Hepper and Shahidullah, 1994) has resulted in most attention being afforded to the fetus's response to sound. Changes in fetal heart rate (Gagnon, 1989; Read and Miller, 1977), movement (Birnholz and Benacerraf, 1983; Shahidullah and Hepper, 1993a) and behavioural state (Devoe, Murray, Faircloth and Ramos, 1990; Visser, Mulder, Witt et al., 1989) have all been observed following presentation of a sound. The fetus first responds to sound at 20 weeks' GA (Shahidullah and Hepper, 1993a). The first responses are to low-frequency sounds (250–500 Hz) of the adult hearing range (20–20 000 Hz) and, as the fetus matures, the range of frequencies responded to expands (Hepper and Shahidullah, 1994). Further, the hearing of the fetus becomes more sensitive with advancing gestational age (Hepper and Shahidullah, 1994). At 25 weeks' GA a sound must be 20–30 dB louder to elicit a response than at 35 weeks' GA. During the final weeks of pregnancy, the fetus is able to discriminate between different sounds (Lecanuet, Granier-Deferre, Jacquet et al., 1993; Shahidullah and Hepper, 1994).

The auditory environment of the fetus is not one of silence, but rather one of continual changing sound (Hepper and Shahidullah, 1994; Querleu, Renard,

Boutteville and Crepin, 1989). Internal sounds from the mother's heartbeat, digestive system and borborgymi (gas rumbling in the intestine) will be present throughout pregnancy (Querleu, Renard and Crepin, 1981). External sounds will also be present in the fetal environment (Querleu, Renard, Versyp et al., 1988). The mother's voice clearly emerges above the internal noise of the maternal abdomen and thus may be heard by the fetus (Querleu, Renard, Versyp et al., 1988). Sounds from the external environment are attenuated by the maternal abdomen before reaching the fetus. High-frequency components of the sound (above 1000 Hz) will be greatly reduced in intensity, thus sound *in utero* will 'sound' appreciably different than when heard *ex utero* (Hepper and Shahidullah, 1994).

Chemosensation

Olfactory and gustatory senses are considered together as it is difficult to separate the two *in utero* since both receptor types may be stimulated by chemical stimuli present in the amniotic fluid. De Snoo (1937) reported that the fetus has a 'sweet tooth' observing increased swallowing when saccharin was added to the amniotic fluid. Furthermore, a decrease in sucking was observed when a noxious substance, lipiodol (iodinated poppy seed oil), was added to the amniotic fluid (Liley, 1972). More recently Schaal and Orgeur (1992) report that a newborn infant showed a change in heart rate to an odour, cumin, experienced only *in utero* (added to the maternal diet in the last 12 days of pregnancy).

The fetal environment is rich in chemosensory stimuli. Of chemicals present in the amniotic fluid, lactic and citric acids, fatty acids, uric acids and amino acids are most likely to stimulate chemosensory receptors. Chemical stimuli present in the amniotic fluid are derived from both the mother, via the placenta, and from the fetus, its urine and sebaceous secretion. Thus the fetus's chemosensory environment is one of continual turnover in its constitution (Schaal and Orgeur, 1992).

Cutaneous

Pain

Increases in heart rate have been observed in fetuses following fetal scalp blood sampling and increases in movement have been observed after tactile stimulation during amniocentesis (Hill, Platt and Manning, 1979; Ron, Yaffe and Polishuk, 1976). These are responses which, in adults, may be considered appropriate for a response to pain. The physiological and pharmacological systems responsible for the sensation of pain are present during late gestation (Anand and Hickey, 1987). However it is difficult to determine whether pain is felt by the human fetus since pain is a subjective phenomenon. It is clear that the fetus responds to stimuli that may be viewed as painful in the adult but the observation of a reaction does not imply the fetus feels pain. If a 'painful' stimulus is applied to the foot of a paraplegic one may observe the withdrawal of the foot as if in pain but the individual feels no pain. In the normal course of pregnancy painful stimuli are unlikely to be experienced by the fetus.

Temperature

Anecdotal reports claim that mothers perceive an increase in fetal movements whilst sitting in a hot bath. A jet of cold water, 4°C, squirted at the face of the fetus during labour resulted in a change in fetal heart rate (Timor-Tritsch, 1986). Whether this response is due to temperature or pressure sensation is unknown. The uterine environment is carefully controlled and maintained at 0.5–1.5°C above that of the mother, thus in the normal course of pregnancy there will be little variation in the temperature experienced by the fetus (Walker, 1969).

Touch
The tactile sense is the first sense to be observed functioning prenatally, the first response being observed to a touch on the lips at 8 weeks' GA (Hooker, 1952). By 14 weeks' GA most of the body, excluding the back and top of the head, is responsive to touch. The fetus will be continually stimulated with tactile stimuli during pregnancy; contact with the umbilical cord, the uterine wall, and itself provide varied sources of tactile information.

Proprioception
The fetus exhibits a 'righting reflex' from around 25 weeks' GA. The fact that the fetus attempts to return to its original position in space when the mother changes her position, and hence that of the fetus, is suggestive of a functioning vestibular sense (Hooker, 1952). The observation that the fetus develops a preferred position to lie in may reflect the functioning of the kinaesthetic system. The fact that both the mother and fetus move during the course of pregnancy means that both senses, vestibular and kinaesthetic, will be actively stimulated.

Vision

The visual sense is probably the least likely to be stimulated naturally during the normal course of pregnancy (Hepper, 1992a). Under experimental circumstances presentation of a bright light results in changes in heart rate (Peleg and Goldman, 1980) and movements (Polishuk, Laufer and Sadovsky, 1975) from 26 weeks' GA.

Summary

The fetus's sensory systems are functioning *in utero* with responses exhibited to auditory, cutaneous, chemosensory and visual stimuli. The fetus will experience a diverse and changing array of naturally occurring stimuli (auditory, cutaneous and chemosensory) providing a source of stimulation for the functioning sensory system.

Learning

There have been many experimental demonstrations of learning before birth, in animals (Hepper, 1992b). Indeed for virtually all animal groups there is evidence that individuals before birth, hatching or emergence can learn, e.g. mammals (Hepper, 1988a; Smotherman and Robinson, 1992), birds (Shindler, 1984), amphibians (Hepper and Waldman, 1992) and invertebrates (Caubet, Jaisson and Lenoir, 1992). Given this evidence it is not surprising that studies have sought evidence of learning in the human fetus. However, of all fetal abilities, the ability to learn has been the most controversial and hotly-contested. Part of this is due to the fact that early evidence was largely anecdotal or based on poorly controlled studies and the methodology could not substantiate the reported claims of prenatal learning. In part also, however, there was a reluctance to accept that such an immature organism, the fetus, is capable of learning, one of the pinnacles of adult behavioural and psychological functioning.

The first scientific study of learning in the human fetus was reported by Peiper (1925). He sounded a 'loud and shrill' car horn a few feet away from the abdomen of a pregnant mother during the last few weeks of her pregnancy. On the initial presentations there was a large and marked response by the fetus, however as the stimulus was repeated the response exhibited by the fetus decreased until eventually no response was observed when the horn was sounded, thus demonstrating habituation in the fetus.

Habituation

Since the initial demonstration by Peiper (1925) a number of studies have demonstrated habituation in the fetus. Fetal body movement (e.g. Leader, Baille, Martin and Vermeulen, 1982a) and fetal heart rate (e.g. Lecanuet, Granier-Deferre and Busnel, 1989) habituate to the presentation of an auditory stimulus. In developmental terms habituation has been observed from 23 weeks' GA and it is first observed in females (Leader, Baille, Martin et al., 1984).

Classical conditioning

Few studies have attempted to classically condition the human fetus. Ray (1932) paired a loud sound, the UCS (unconditioned stimulus), with a vibration made by an electric bell-striker hitting on a wooden plate, the CS (conditioned stimulus). Although Ray reports no data in his paper, the last line of the paper states that the subject has 'so far, shown no ill-effects from her prenatal education'. Spelt (1948) repeated the experiment using a loud noise from a wooden clapper as the UCS paired with a vibration produced by a door-bell as the CS. He reports successful conditioning following 15–20 pairings during the last two months of pregnancy. More recently Feijoo (1975, 1981) conditioned fetuses by pairing relaxation, the UCS, with a 12 second burst of music, the CS. After conditioning, presentation of the sound stimulus (CS alone) resulted in a reduced latency of fetal movements. Conditioning was evident after birth where the newborn stopped crying and reduced the incidence of clonic movements upon presentation of the CS.

Exposure learning

A number of studies have examined the effects of simply exposing the fetus to a stimulus, usually auditory, on the fetus's or newborn's subsequent response to that stimulus. Here a differential response to the familiar (experienced prenatally) and unfamiliar (not experienced prenatally) stimulus is taken as evidence of learning.

The newborn infant prefers the voice of its mother over that of an unfamiliar female (DeCasper and Fifer, 1980; DeCasper and Prescott, 1984). Furthermore newborns prefer their mother's voice as it sounds in utero over their mother's voice as it sound ex utero, indicating the preference is acquired prenatally (Fifer and Moon, 1989). Salk (1960, 1962) found that newborns played the sound of a heartbeat at 72 bpm during the first few days following birth gained more weight and cried less than those who did not hear the heartbeat sound. Infants at 16–37 months of age, when played the sound of the hearbeat fell asleep faster than those not played the sound of a heartbeat. Although it has been argued that this is the result of prenatal familiarization with the maternal heartbeat sound *in utero*, it is unclear whether these effects are due to prenatal learning or a genetic preference (Hepper, 1989). Hepper (1988b, 1991) found that newborn infants of mothers who had watched a particular TV 'soap' opera during pregnancy stopped crying, became alert and exhibited a change in both heart rate and movements when played that tune, but not unfamiliar tunes, after birth. A differential response, increased movement, was observed to the familiar tune at 36 weeks' GA but not 30 weeks' GA, which may suggest experience of the tune in the last trimester of pregnancy is important for subsequent recognition (Hepper, 1991).

Summary

The ability of the fetus to learn suggests other abilities are also present. Differential responding to familiar and unfamiliar tunes implies some form of discrimination ability in the fetus. The success of classical conditioning paradigms suggests the fetus possesses the ability to form associations. Finally the exhibition of a response to a previously experienced stimulus implies the fetus also possesses a memory.

Functions of fetal behaviour

The behaviours evidenced during the prenatal period may serve a number of functions for the current and future development of the individual. Some of these are briefly described below.

However, it is appropriate at this stage to introduce a note of caution when interpreting the behaviour of the fetus. Although a number of fetal abilities have been demonstrated, care must be taken before inferring direct comparability with similar behaviours exhibited after birth. Whether similar prenatal and postnatal behaviours represent the same ability or are mediated by the same physiological, anatomical or pharmacological structures needs careful consideration. A good illustration of this is the observation of rapid eye movements. Rapid eye movements in adults are associated with deep sleep and dreaming and may serve a number of different functions (Horne, 1983). However, is it possible for a fetus to dream? If it does dream, what does it dream about? Great care must be exercised in interpreting fetal behavioural patterns in terms of adult functions.

Neural development

It is now recognized that the development and structure of the nervous system is not purely the result of genetic instructions but rather reflects an interaction between genetic and environmental influences (Greenough, Black and Wallace, 1987). Electrical activity within the nervous system may influence its development and structure (Purves, 1994). Thus neural activity generated by the motor behaviour of the fetus may structure the motor nervous system (Purves and Lichtman, 1985) whilst neural activity generated by the reception of sensory stimuli may influence sensory neural structure (Hirsch and Spinelli, 1970). Although the outside world (of the brain) does not directly influence brain development, the electrical activity generated within the nervous system by the fetus's motor behaviour or the reception of sensory stimuli does influence brain growth. The activity generated within the fetus's nervous system by its movements (starting at 7 weeks' GA) and by the reception of sensory stimuli (auditory, visual, cutaneous, olfactory and gustatory stimuli are present throughout the fetus's period in the womb) will be expected to exert an influence on the development and structure of the CNS. Although the evidence is very limited in the prenatal period, there is much evidence after birth that neural activity is essential for the normal development of the brain. The classic studies here were performed by Hubel and Weisel (see review by Hubel, 1988) where they demonstrated that normal visual stimulation was necessary for the development of the visual cortex (Hubel and Weisel, 1963). More recently the development of the somatic sensory cortex has been shown to be influenced by neural activity (Riddle, Gutierrez, Zheng et al., 1993). Thus normal fetal behaviour may play an important role in developing the individual's nervous system.

Anatomical structure

The motor behaviour of the fetus is essential for the normal development of the limbs and joints (Moessinger, 1988). Restrictions of movements of a particular joint *in utero* may result in an abnormality of that limb, primarily the result of joint cavities becoming filled with connective tissue making the joint rigid (Drachman and Sokoloff, 1966). Joint deformities in newborns arising from genetic conditions, e.g. Pena–Shokeir syndrome, may be due to fetal immobilization *in utero* (Hall, 1986).

Language

The acquisition of language may commence in the womb. The mother's voice, and other voices, can be clearly 'heard' by the fetus above the background noise present in its uterine environment (Querleu, Renard, Versyp et al., 1988). Although the abdomen differentially attenuates different frequencies (Querleu, Renard, Boutteville and Crepin, 1989) the prosodic elements of speech, i.e. the intonation, stress and rhythm of language are largely unaffected by this and will be experienced unaltered by the fetus. Infants pay attention to the prosodic elements of speech and this may have arisen from prenatal experience, and may form the beginnings of language acquisition (Fifer and Moon, 1989).

Breast feeding

The establishment of breast feeding may be promoted by chemosensory learning in the womb. The maternal diet influences the sensory characteristics of breast milk (Mennella and Beauchamp, 1991) and amniotic fluid (Nolte, Provenza, Callan and Panter, 1992). Mothers who had maintained their diet before and after birth were much more successful in initiating breast feeding and their infants took more food than the mothers who had changed their diet from before to after birth (Hepper, unpublished observations). The fetus initially experiences the diet of its mother in the amniotic fluid and later, when born, in the breast milk. Mothers eating the same diet before and after birth 'flavour' their amniotic fluid and breast milk similarly. The newborn is thus familiar with the 'taste' of the breast milk through previous exposure as a fetus *in utero* and thus readily sucks and ingests the breast milk. Where mothers change their diet, eating a different diet, before and after birth the newborn is unfamiliar with the 'flavour' of its mother's breast milk and may not suck so readily in the absence of prenatal experiences with the 'flavour' in the amniotic fluid.

Maternal recognition

Newborns have been demonstrated to recognize their mother's voice immediately following birth (e.g. DeCasper and Fifer, 1980) and this may be important for the establishment of maternal recognition. Newborns also recognize their mother's odour soon after birth (Porter, 1991), an ability which may be acquired prenatally (Hepper, 1992a). Both may prime the newborn to recognize the mother immediately after birth.

Clinical applications

A description of normal fetal behaviour may be used as a standard against which the behaviour of individual fetuses may be compared to assess the normal progression of development and functioning (Hepper, 1990). The use of fetal behaviour as a means of assessing neural system functioning has proved possible. All aspects of the fetus's behaviour have been used to assess well-being and three examples are presented below to illustrate how the motor, sensory and learning behaviour of the fetus may be used.

Observations of the direction of fetal eye movements revealed this could be used to indicate the presence of the genetic disorder, Edwards syndrome, Trisomy 18 (Hepper and Shahidullah, 1992a). In normal fetuses the majority of single eye movements (78%) are in the horizontal plane whereas for a fetus with Trisomy 18, the majority (69%) are in the vertical plane. Thus the spontaneous behaviour of the fetus, in this case eye movements, can indicate the presence of an abnormality in the individual's neural system.

The fact that the fetus responds to sound was used to develop a tool to diagnose deafness prenatally (Shahidullah and Hepper, 1993b). By presenting a series of sounds (via a headphone placed on the mother's abdomen) and light (a cold halogen light shone on the mother's abdomen) it was possible to differentiate fetuses who were deaf (responded to the light but not the sound) from fetuses in a non-responsive behavioural state (did not respond to either sound or light) from those who could hear (responded to light and sound). The prenatal recognition of deafness enables alternative communication strategies to be adopted from the moment of birth compensating for the newborn's inability to hear.

Finally one technique which has proved most promising in assessing neural system function is that of habituation (Hepper and Shahidullah, 1992b). Differences in habituation patterns have been noted in microcephalics, anencephalics, individuals with meconium staining and low birth weight individuals (Leader, Baille, Martin and Vermeulen, 1982b; Leader, Baille, Martin et al., 1984). Habituation patterns not only distinguish Down's syndrome individuals from unaffected individuals but also enables the severity of Down's syndrome to be determined (Hepper and Shahidullah, 1992b) marking a significant advance in our ability to determine fetal health.

Summary

The ultimate arbitor of well-being is the functioning and integrity of the nervous system. Since the behaviour of the fetus directly reflects the integrity of the CNS, the behaviour of the fetus can be used to assess its well-being. The detailed study of the behaviour of the fetus promises significant advances in the ability to determine the health of the fetus.

Ethical implications

As more information is obtained regarding the behavioural development of the fetus, and its abilities, this may be used to inform ethical issues regarding the treatment of the fetus. No attempt is made here to solve these ethical 'problems' but rather to indicate areas where such information may be usefully applied.

The presence of certain abilities may have relevance for issues which involve a time limit. Determining the upper limit for abortions or the period during which research on embryos may take place may well be influenced by the presence or absence of particular abilities.

The question of pain in the newborn has been a topic of some concern (e.g. Anand and Hickey, 1987) and with advances in techniques which enable surgery to be undertaken on the fetus (Evans, Adzick, Johnson et al., 1994) the question of appropriate pain relief in the fetus is now pertinent.

One area of great ethical complexity concerns potential maternal–fetal conflict. It is now generally accepted that the development of fetal behavioural abilities results from an interaction between the individual's genes and environment. Alterations in either of these may result in adverse effects on the developing individual. The effects of genetic or chromosomal abnormalities are well known, but of more interest are the effects of environmental agents, in particular those with the potential for abuse by the mother, e.g. alcohol and drugs. Here low-level exposure to these substances may effect the functioning of the CNS, resulting in behavioural, educational and social problems, but not gross physical anomalies, which may arise with higher levels of exposure. Questions may then be raised regarding what course of action to take if the mother acts in a fashion potentially damaging to the normal development of the fetus, e.g. continues drinking or smoking when pregnant. The situation greatly increases in complexity with the appreciation that maternal stress may adversely affect the development of the fetus (van den Bergh, 1992). Actions taken to limit maternal behaviours with the aim of benefiting the fetus, i.e. reducing alcohol intake, may increase stress.

A greater understanding of the prenatal development process may contribute to the debate on ethical consideration of the fetus. However it should be born in mind that the behavioural abilities of the fetus should be interpreted in context. Although it is tempting to directly equate fetal abilities with those of the human adult it must be recognized that all of the abilities demonstrated in the human fetus have also been demonstrated in other animal groups, including learning in invertebrate pupae, e.g. ants and wasps (Caubet, Jaisson and Lenoir, 1992).

Conclusion

Scientific study of human behavioural ontogenesis shows the fetus possesses a sophisticated repertoire of behaviour that enables it to respond to its changing environment. The fetus is neither a passive organism developing in sensory isolation nor a fully sentient conscious mini-adult experiencing all the sensations of an adult. A more appropriate view of the fetus is that it is an extremely well adapted individual suited uniquely to the environment in which it develops. The environment of the fetus has evolved to ensure that the fetus receives the appropriate stimulation to promote normal development. The behaviour of the fetus is structured to make maximum use of the stimulation present in its environment. The fetus's biological make-up combines and interacts with its environment to ensure development proceeds along its normal course.

Much more work is needed to fully unravel behavioural development during the prenatal period. This is important for itself and for advances in other areas as mentioned above. The careful observation and description of fetal behaviour will provide the basis for answering questions about the earliest stages of human psychological development.

Applications

1. The care of very pre-term babies may be improved by applying the knowledge gained from the study of the fetus of the same conceptual age. Such improvements may enable survival at an earlier gestational age, or may benefit the babies' quality of life.

2. New techniques for assessing fetal health can be developed based on information about normal behaviour patterns and responses in the fetus. For example, the analysis of movement in the fetus suggests that some individual differences are apparent, which may be related to their survivability.

Acknowledgements

I thank the Wellcome Trust and the Medical Research Council for their support.

Further reading

Nathanielsz, P. (1992). *Life before birth and a time to be born.* New York: Promethean.
Nijhuis, J. G. (ed.) (1992). *Fetal behaviour. Developmental and perinatal aspects.* Oxford: Oxford University Press.
Smotherman, W. P. and Robinson, S. R. (eds) (1988). *The behavior of the fetus.* New Jersey: Telford.

References

Anand, K. J. S. and Hickey, P. R. (1987). Pain and its effects in the human neonate and fetus. *New England Journal of Medicine*, **317**, 1321–9.

Birnholz, J. C. (1981). The development of human fetal eye movements. *Science*, **213**, 679–81.

Birnholz, J. C. and Benacerraf, B. R. (1983). The development of human fetal hearing. *Science*, **222**, 516–18.

Birnholz, J. C., Stephens, J. C. and Faria, M. (1978). Fetal movement patterns: A possible means of defining neurologic developmental milestones in utero. *American Journal of Roentgenology*, **130**, 537–40.

Caubet, Y., Jaisson, P. and Lenoir, A. (1992). Preimaginal induction of adult behaviour in insects. *Quarterly Journal of Experimental Psychology*, **44B**, 165–78.

DeCasper, A. J. and Fifer, W. P. (1980). Of human bonding: Newborns prefer their mothers' voices. *Science*, **208**, 1174–6.

DeCasper, A. J. and Prescott, P. A. (1984). Human newborns' perception of male voices: Preference, discrimination and reinforcing value. *Developmental Psychobiology*, **17**, 481–91.

De Snoo, K. (1937). Das trinkende Kind im Uterus. *Monatsschr. Geburtsh. Gynaekol.*, **105**, 88–97.

Devoe, L. D., Murray, C., Faircloth, D. and Ramos, E. (1990). Vibroacoustic stimulation and fetal behavioural state in normal and term human pregnancy. *American Journal of Obstetrics and Gynecology*, **163**, 1156–61.

Dewbury, K., Meire, H. and Cosgrove, D. (1993). *Ultrasound in obstetrics and gynaecology.* Edinburgh: Churchill Livingstone.

Diamond, A. (1990). The development and neural basis of higher cognitive function. *Annals of the New York Academy of Science*, **608**, 1–751.

Drachman, D. B. and Sokoloff, L. (1966). The role of movement in embryonic joint development. *Developmental Biology*, **14**, 401–20.

Ellis, H. (1940). *Studies in the psychology of sex.* New York: Random House.

Evans, M. I., Adzick, N. S., Johnson, M. P., Flake, A. W., Quintero, R. and Harrison, M. R. (1994). Fetal therapy – 1994. *Current Opinion in Obstetrics and Gynecology*, **6**, 58–64.

Feijoo, J. (1975). Ut Conscientia Noscatue. *Cahier de Sophrologie*, **13**, 14–20.

Feijoo, J. (1981). Le foetus Pierre et le loup ... ou une approche originale de l'audition prenatale humaine. In *L'aube des Sens* (E. Herbinet and M. C. Busnel, eds). Paris: Stock.

Fifer, W. P. and Moon, C. (1989). Psychobiology of newborn auditory preferences. *Seminars in Perinatology*, **13**, 430–3.

Gagnon, R. (1989). Stimulation of human fetuses with sound and vibration. *Seminars in Perinatology*, **13**, 393–402.

Greenough, W. T., Black, J. E. and Wallace, C. S. (1987). Experience and brain development. *Child Development*, **58**, 539–59.

Hall, J. G. (1986). Analysis of the Pena Shokeir phenotype. *American Journal of Medical Genetics*, **25**, 99–117.

Hepper, P. G. (1988a). Adaptive fetal learning: prenatal exposure to garlic affects postnatal preferences. *Animal Behaviour*, **36**, 935–6.

Hepper, P. G. (1988b). Foetal 'soap' addiction. *The Lancet*, 11 June, 1347–8.

Hepper, P. G. (1989). Foetal learning: Implications for Psychiatry? *British Journal of Psychiatry*, **155**, 289–93.

Hepper, P. G. (1990). Diagnosing handicap using the behaviour of the fetus. *Midwifery*, **6**, 193–200.

Hepper, P. G. (1991). An examination of fetal learning before and after birth. *Irish Journal of Psychology*, **12**, 95–107.

Hepper, P. G. (1992a). Fetal psychology. An embryonic science. In *Fetal behaviour. Developmental and perinatal aspects* (J. G. Nijhuis, ed.). Oxford: Oxford University Press.

Hepper, P. G. (ed.) (1992b). *Comparative studies of prenatal learning and behaviour.* London: LEA.

Hepper, P. G. and Shahidullah, S. (1992a). Trisomy 18: behavioral and structural abnormalities. An ultrasonographic case study. *Ultrasound in Obstetrics and Gynecology*, **2**, 48–50.

Hepper, P. G. and Shahidullah, S. (1992b). Habituation in normal and Down Syndrome fetuses. *Quarterly Journal of Experimental Psychology*, **44B**, 305–17.

Hepper, P. G. and Shahidullah, S. (1994). *Noise and the foetus.* Sudbury: HSE Books.

Hepper, P. G. and Shahidullah, S. (1994). Development of fetal hearing. *Archives of Disease in Childhood*, **71**, F81–F87.

Hepper, P. G. and Waldman, B. (1992). Embryonic learning in an amphibian. *Quarterly Journal of Experimental Psychology*, **44B**, 179–96.

Hill, L. M., Platt, L. D. and Manning, F. A. (1979). Immediate effects of amniocentesis on fetal breathing and gross body movements. *American Journal of Obstetrics and Gynecology*, **135**, 689–90.

Hirsch, H. V. B. and Spinelli, D. N. (1970). Visual experience modifies distribution of horizontally and vertically oriented receptive fields in cats. *Science*, **168**, 869–71.

Hooker, D. (1952). *The prenatal origin of behaviour.* Kansas: University of Kansas Press.

Horimoto, N., Hepper, P. G., Shahidullah, S. and Koyanagi, T. (1993). Fetal eye movements. *Ultrasound in Obstetrics and Gynecology*, **3**, 362–9.

Horne, J. A. (1983). Mammalian sleep function with particular reference to man. In *Sleep mechanisms and functions in humans and animals* (A. R. Mayes, ed.). Wokingham: Van Nostrand Reinhold.

Hubel, D. H. (1988). *Eye, brain and vision.* New York: W. H. Freeman.

Hubel, D. H. and Weisel, T. N. (1963). Receptive fields of cells in the striate cortex of very young, visually inexperienced kittens. *Journal of Neurophysiology*, **26**, 994–1002.

Humphrey, T. (1978). Function of the nervous system during prenatal life. In *Perinatal physiology* (U. Stave, ed.). New York: Plenum.

Ianniruberto, A. and Tajani, E. (1981). Ultrasonic study of fetal movements. *Seminars in Perinatology*, **5**, 175–81.

Leader, L. R., Baille, P., Martin, B., Molteno, C. and Wynchank, S. (1984). Foetal responses to vibrotactile stimulation. A possible predictor of foetal and neonatal outcome. *Australian and New Zealand Journal of Obstetrics and Gynaecology*, **24**, 251–6.

Leader, L. R., Baille, P., Martin, B. and Vermeulen, E. (1982a). The assessment and significance of habituation to a repeated stimulus by the human foetus. *Early Human Development*, **7**, 211–19.

Leader, L. R., Baille, P., Martin, B. and Vermeulen, E. (1982b). Foetal habituation in high risk pregnancies. *British Journal of Obstetrics and Gynaecology*, **89**, 441–6.

Lecanuet, J-P., Granier-Deferre, C. and Busnel, M-C. (1989). Differential auditory reactiveness as a function of stimulus characteristics and state. *Seminars in Perinatology*, **13**, 421–9.

Lecanuet, J-P., Granier-Deferre, C., Jacquet, A. Y., Capponi, I. and Ledru, L. (1993). Prenatal discrimination of a male and female voice uttering the same sentence. *Early Development and Parenting*, **2**, 217–28.

Liley, A. W. (1972). The foetus as a personality. *Australian and New Zealand Journal of Psychiatry*, **6**, 99–105.

Mennella, J. A. and Beauchamp, G. K. (1991). Maternal diet alters the sensory qualities of human milk and the nurslings behavior. *Pediatrics*, **88**, 737–44.

Minkowski, M. (1928). Neurobiologische studien am menschlichen foetus. *Handbk biol. ArbMeth*, **5**, 511–618.

Moessinger, A. C. (1988). Morphological consequences of depressed or impaired fetal activity. In *Behavior of the fetus* (W. P. Smotherman and S. R. Robson, eds). New Jersey: Telford.

Nijhuis, J. G. (1986). Behavioral states: concomitants, clinical implications and the assessment of the condition of the nervous system. *European Journal of Obstetrics, Gynecology and Reproductive Biology*, **21**, 301–8.

Nijhuis, J. G., Prechtl, H. F. R., Martin, C. B. and Bots, R. S. G. M. (1982). Are there behavioural states in the human fetus? *Early Human Development*, **6**, 177–95.

Nolte, D. L., Provenza, F. D., Callan, R. and Panter, K. E. (1992). Garlic in the ovine fetal environment. *Physiology and Behavior*, **52**, 1091–3.

Patrick, J., Campbell, K., Carmichael, L., Natale, R. and Richardson, B. (1980). Patterns of human fetal breathing during the last 10 weeks of pregnancy. *Obstetrics and Gynecology*, **56**, 24–30.

Peiper, A. (1925). Sinnesempfindungen des Kindes vor seiner geburt. *Monatsschrift fur Kinderheilkunde*, **29**, 237–41.

Peleg, D. and Goldman, J. A. (1980). Fetal heart rate acceleration in response to light stimulation as a clinical measure of fetal well-being. A preliminary report. *Journal of Perinatal Medicine*, **8**, 38–41.

Pillai, M. and James, D. (1990). Behavioural states in normal mature human fetuses. *Archives of Disease in Childhood*, **65**, 39–43.

Pillai, M., James, D. K. and Parker, M. (1992). The development of ultradian rhythms in the human fetus. *American Journal of Obstetrics and Gynecology*, **167**, 172–7.

Polishuk, W. Z., Laufer, N. and Sadovsky, E. (1975). Fetal reaction to external light. *Harefuah*, **89**, 395–7.

Porter, R. H. (1991). Mutual mother–infant recognition in humans. In *Kin recognition* (P. G. Hepper, ed.). Cambridge: Cambridge University Press.

Prechtl, H. F. R. (1974). The behavioural states of the newborn infant (a review). *Brain Research*, **76**, 1304–11.

Prechtl, H. F. R. and Beintema, D. J. (1964). The neurological examination of the full term newborn infant. *Clinics in Developmental Medicine*, **12**. London: Heinmann.

Preyer, W. (1885). *Die spezielle physiologie des embryo*. Leipzig: Grieben.

Purves, D. (1994). *Neural activity and the growth of the brain*. Cambridge: Cambridge University Press.

Purves, D. and Lichtman, J. W. (1985). *Principles of neural development*. Sunderland, MA: Sinauer Assoc.

Querleu, D., Renard, X. and Crepin, G. (1981). Bruit intra-uterin et perceptions auditives du foetus. *Bulletin Academie Nationale de Medecine*, **165**, 581–8.

Querleu, D., Renard, X., Boutteville, C. and Crepin, G. (1989). Hearing by the human fetus? *Seminars in Perinatology*, **13**, 409–20.

Querleu, D., Renard, X., Versyp, F., Paris-Delrue, L. and Crepin, G. (1988). Fetal hearing. *European Journal of Obstetrics, Gynecology and Reproductive Biology*, **29**, 191–212.

Ray, W. S. (1932). A preliminary report on a study of foetal conditioning. *Child Development*, **3**, 175–7.

Read, J. and Miller, F. (1977). Fetal heart rate acceleration in response to acoustic stimulation as a measure of fetal well-being. *American Journal of Obstetrics and Gynecology*, **129**, 512–17.

Reinold, E. (1971). Beobachtung foetaler Aktivitat in der ersten Halfte der graviditat mit dem ultraschall. *Padiatrie und Padologie*, **6**, 274–9.

Riddle, D. R., Gutierrez, G., Zheng, D., White, L., Richards, A. and Purves, D. (1993). Differential metabolic and electrical activity in the somatic sensory cortex of the developing rat. *Journal of Neuroscience*, **13**, 4193–213.

Ron, M., Yaffe, H. and Polishuk, W. Z. (1976). Fetal heart rate response to amniocentesis in cases of decreased fetal movements. *Obstetrics and Gynecology*, **48**, 456–9.

Salk, L. (1960). The effects of the normal heartbeat sound on the behaviour of the new-born infant: Implications for mental health. *World Mental Health*, **12**, 168–75.

Salk, L. (1962). Mothers' heartbeat as an imprinting stimulus. *Transactions of the New York Academy of Science*, **24**, 753–63.

Schaal, B. and Orgeur, P. (1992). Olfaction in utero. Can the rodent model be generalised? *Quarterly Journal of Experimental Psychology*, **44B**, 245–78.

Shahidullah, S. and Hepper, P. G. (1993a). The developmental origins of fetal responsiveness to an acoustic stimulus. *Journal of Reproductive and Infant Psychology*, **11**, 135–42.

Shahidullah, S. and Hepper, P. G. (1993b). Prenatal hearing tests? *Journal of Reproductive and Infant Psychology*, **11**, 143–6.

Shahidullah, S. and Hepper, P. G. (1994). Frequency discrimination by the fetus. *Early Human Development*, **36**, 13–26.

Shindler, K. M. (1984). A three year study of fetal auditory imprinting. *Journal of the Washington Academy of Science*, **74**, 121–4.

Smotherman, W. P. and Robinson, S. R. (1992). Habituation in the rat fetus. *Quarterly Journal of Experimental Psychology*, **44B**, 215–30.

Spelt, D. K. (1948). The conditioning of the human foetus in utero. *Journal of Experimental Psychology*, **38**, 338–46.

Timor-Tritsch, I. E. (1986). The effect of external stimuli on fetal behaviour. *European Journal of Obstetrics, Gynecology and Reproductive Biology*, **21**, 321–9.

van den Bergh, B. R. H. (1992). Maternal emotions during pregnancy and fetal and neonatal behaviour. In *Fetal behaviour* (J. G. Nijhuis, ed.). 157–78. Oxford: Oxford University Press.

van Dongen, L. G. R. and Goudie, E. G. (1980). Fetal movement patterns in the first trimester of pregnancy. *British Journal of Obstetrics and Gynaecology*, **87**, 191–3.

Visser, G. H. A., Mulder, H. H., Wit, H. P., Mulder, E. J. H. and Prechtl, H. F. R. (1989). Vibro-acoustic stimulation of the human fetus: effect on behavioural state organisation. *Early Human Development*, **19**, 285–96.

de Vries, J. I. P., Visser, G. H. A. and Prechtl, H. F. R. (1982). The emergence of fetal behaviour I Qualitative aspects. *Early Human Development*, **7**, 301–22.

de Vries, J. I. P., Visser, G. H. A. and Prechtl, H. F. R. (1985). The emergence of fetal behaviour II Qualitative aspects. *Early Human Development*, **12**, 99–120.

de Vries, J. I. P., Visser, G. H. A. and Prechtl, H. F. R. (1988). The emergence of fetal behaviour III Individual differences and consistencies. *Early Human Development*, **16**, 85–103.

Walker, D. (1969). Temperature of the human fetus. *Journal of Obstetrics and Gynaecology of the British Commonwealth*, **76**, 503–11.

6

Prenatal screening

Jenny Hewison

> The growth of prenatal screening has altered the experience of pregnancy for women in medicalized societies, as Chapter 4 discussed. In this chapter, Jenny Hewison points out the physical and psychological costs and benefits attached to prenatal screening and discusses the ethical dilemmas that this raises. While screening of all sorts, e.g. for cancer, carries the same dual potential to cause and (when negative) relieve anxiety, few other forms carry the risks that invasive prenatal testing has – that of causing the death of the fetus through miscarriage. Nor do they offer such little hope of treating the problem uncovered by positive test results. The need for more and better psychological input is clear.

Detecting abnormalities in the fetus is an important part of antenatal care, intended to increase the reproductive choices available to women. The drawbacks of increased choice however is that pregnant women nowadays face many complex and difficult decisions. The availability of powerful techniques of prenatal diagnosis and selective abortion mean that large numbers of people are faced with explicit life and death choices. Few people – users or providers of health care – will be faced with decisions as stark as these in any other aspect of their lives.

Confronting these decisions would be difficult enough if they were clear cut. Unfortunately, even though technological development is very rapid, the goal of risk-free, affordable and conclusive diagnostic testing has not yet been reached. The two main diagnostic tests which are available for chromosomal abnormalities both require samples of fetal cells. These samples have to be obtained by invasive means, which increases the risk of miscarriage, and possibly of damage to the fetus. For many women, the risk of a procedure-induced miscarriage exceeds that of having an affected child, so some other approach is required.

The approach currently adopted is to try and find ways of identifying subgroups of women for whom the balance tilts the other way, i.e. women who are at significantly increased risk of carrying an abnormal fetus. Invasive diagnostic testing is then only offered to these subgroups. Screening for Down's syndrome follows this pattern. Because it is widely available, and because its underlying logic exemplifies the approach currently taken to the development of screening tests, it is used to illustrate many of the points in this chapter. Screening for neural tube defects, such as spina bifida, follows a similar logic, and is even more widely available. Carrier screening for genetic disorders such as cystic fibrosis is likely to be the biggest growth area in the future. It is discussed in a separate section towards the end of the chapter.

Subgroups 'at risk' for a particular condition may be defined on the basis of readily ascertainable information, such as maternal age or family history, or on the basis of screening test results. Biochemical screening tests are based on established relationships between the levels of certain chemicals in the mother's blood and an increased risk of abnormality in the fetus. Ultrasound screening relies on relationships between features measurable on the scan, and the probability of abnormality. Combining information from different 'markers' increases the accuracy of screening. The 'triple test' for Down's syndrome is based on the mathematical combination of information about maternal age plus three serum markers: raised maternal serum human chorionic gonadotrophin (hCG), low maternal serum unconjugated oestriol (uE3), and low maternal serum alphafetoprotein (AFP) (Wald, Cuckle, Densem et al., 1988). In addition, information about the length of gestation is necessary for the correct calculation of a risk estimate. This estimate represents the probability, based on all the information available, that the fetus in this particular pregnancy has Down's syndrome. If the risk is higher than some prespecified level – usually 1 in 250 or 1 in 300 – and taking into account the woman's own views, then diagnostic testing would be offered.

Here lies the problem. The information from screening tests is by definition probabilistic. Some women who are 'screen positive' (i.e. their calculated risk is high) are in fact carrying normal babies; and some women who are 'screen negative' are in fact carrying a baby with Down's syndrome.

The probability of a designated screen positive result on the triple test increases with maternal age, but is of the order of 5%. The great majority of these are false positives: Reynolds, Nix, Dunstan and Dawson (1993) calculated that with a risk cut-off of 1 : 300, the positive predictive value is about 1% for women under 35, and only 3.8% for a 44 year old. Put another way, for 44 year olds, there will be only one Down's syndrome fetus per 26 screen positive pregnancies. Up to 35 or so, it is about 1/100–110.

On the other side of the coin, serum screening currently detects about 60% of pregnancies with Down's syndrome; the other 40% occur in women with no identifiable risk factor.

The clock cannot be turned back, and the decision whether or not to have Down's screening now faces all pregnant women. The complexity of the task facing them can be summarized as follows. If parents decline testing, they have a risk of having a Down's affected child that varies with the mother's age. If they choose a test, they have three options: an early invasive diagnostic test, chorionic villus biopsy (CVB) with a relatively high risk (2–4%) of causing miscarriage; a late invasive diagnostic test, amniocentesis, with a lower (0.5–1%) risk of miscarriage; or a blood test with no risk of miscarriage. The blood test for Down's syndrome (the triple test) is not diagnostic, but produces a better estimate of risk for that particular pregnancy. Invasive tests are then available if the revised risk exceeds a particular threshold. However, the blood test is performed at 16–18 weeks, which is too late for diagnosis by CVB, and hence, if desired, for termination of pregnancy by early and less traumatic methods.

The position is now becoming even more complicated, with the possibility of first trimester (i.e. in the first three months of pregnancy) ultrasound screening for Down's syndrome. The potential of this approach has been demonstrated in a number of recent studies (for example, Nicolaides, Azar, Byrne et al., 1992; Schulte-Vallentin and Schindler, 1992). Although the technical aspects have not been fully evaluated (screening efficiency may be higher in expert centres and ultrasound may preferentially detect fetuses that are due to miscarry), ultrasound screening is certain to become more widespread. Full technical evaluation of the comparative and of the combined clinical efficiency of ultrasound and serum screening techniques is, however, likely to take some time because of the need to achieve an adequate sample, and because of the low incidence of Down's syndrome in women under 35.

Understanding of risk

All of these screening procedures for Down's syndrome have the same aim, which is to reduce the number of women having to undergo invasive diagnostic testing, at the same time as increasing the number of affected fetuses detected. They also have the same drawbacks, which are basically psychological and educational in nature. Most people find the ideas of probability and of risk difficult to understand. The same risk figure can be perceived as high by one person, and low by another. Actual and perceived risks may be very different (Shiloh and Saxe, 1989), and it is the latter which will influence behaviour (Marteau, Kidd and Cook, 1991).

When applied to whether or not a particular baby has Down's syndrome, an understandable response from a parent to a risk estimate is 'But surely, either it has or it hasn't'. This is in fact correct. The risk estimate given in these circumstances reflects not a risk in the everyday sense of the term (e.g. the risk of being run over when crossing the road), but the experts' degree of uncertainty about an event which has already taken place, at conception, some months before.

Time and skill are required to provide women with all the information they need to make informed choices about prenatal testing, without creating unnecessary anxiety. Even if presented well, screening testing can set in place a series of events and choices which, with hindsight, some women would rather have avoided. Support and counselling may be required at a number of different stages in that chain. Interestingly, the costs of providing counselling and support have usually been overlooked in economic analyses of prenatal screening programmes (e.g. Sheldon and Simpson, 1991). One detailed cost-benefit analysis (Seror, Muller, Moatti et al., 1993) omitted counselling costs for serum screening, although they were included for the small number of women subsequently offered amniocentesis.

The availability of the triple test, and the publicity it has received, have drawn new attention to prenatal testing. Serum screening has, however, been common-place in antenatal clinics for many years, but as a screen for neural tube defects, rather than Down's syndrome. High levels of maternal serum alpha feto-protein (MSAFP) are associated with increased risks of anencephaly and spina bifida; almost all of the former can be identified by screening, and about 85% of the latter. Like the triple test, MSAFP screening has a high false positive rate, i.e. pregnancies where high levels of MSAFP are identified, but where no neural tube defect is found on subsequent ultrasound scanning, and no other anomaly identified by amniocentesis.

Because the triple test has become widely available only in the last few years, most of the research on the psychological implications of prenatal testing has been done in connection with MSAFP screening. It must also be noted that work to date has concentrated almost entirely on implications for women, and very little is known about the contribution of fathers to decisions about prenatal testing or the effects it has upon them.

Uptake and consequences of prenatal screening

Marteau and colleagues studied factors affecting the uptake of MSAFP testing, and found that demographic factors were not related to uptake, but that knowledge of the test and attitudes to termination were related (Marteau, Johnston, Shaw and Slack, 1989a; Johnston and Marteau, 1990). Green and colleagues (1993) studied pregnant women's attitudes to abortion, and noted that although 84% regarded 'a strong chance' of handicap as an acceptable reason for abortion, only 66% said that they themselves would consider terminating a pregnancy for this reason. Twenty-nine per cent of women in this study who had had routine MSAFP testing said that they would not consider termination. Other data suggest however that when a serious abnormality is in fact detected, most women decide to terminate the pregnancy.

Marteau and colleagues (1992a) also compared three psychological models in their ability to predict attendance at prenatal screening: Ley's cognitive hypothesis, which emphasizes the information available to women; 'subjective expected utility theory', which emphasizes beliefs about threats to health; and the 'theory of reasoned action', which in this context emphasizes attitudes towards medicine and doctors. Some support was found for all three theories, but even in combination, they could only explain about a fifth of the variation in uptake behaviour, i.e. their predictive power was quite modest.

In interpreting the above, it must however be noted that MSAFP testing often took place without the women knowing what was being done or why (Faden, Chwalow, Orel-Crosby, 1985; Marteau, Johnston, Plenicar et al., 1988a). In these circumstances, the interpretation of uptake rates must be problematic. One reason advanced for the high uptake rates for MSAFP testing (90% in the Marteau et al., study) is that the test was presented to women as a matter of routine procedure, which they must assert themselves to avoid.

In a review paper, Green, Statham and Snowdon (1992) point out that 'a woman who is ambivalent about the possibility of learning that her baby has an abnormality may still choose to have screening because her need for reassurance takes priority'. They also draw attention to what Tymstra (1989) called 'anticipated decision regret', i.e. the tendency to make a particular choice partly in order to avoid future regret at not having made that choice. These and similar factors are, however, likely to have only a modest role in explaining high levels of uptake of prenatal testing. Rather, it seems that many women do not have sufficient information to make an active decision about testing; and that passive acceptance is encouraged by the way in which testing is offered. Commenting on the reassurance which women gained from MSAFP screening, Green and colleagues (1992) wrote, ' it is quite likely that women would find screening less reassuring if they understood its limitations'.

Problems of interpretation also occur with uptake figures for serum screening for Down's syndrome. In this case, there is considerable variation in uptake rates in different centres. In the study undertaken by Wald, Kennard, Densem et al. (1992), the uptake rate for the triple test was 74%. Evidence from a randomized trial of prenatal counselling (Thornton, Hewison, Lilford and Vail, 1995) suggests that the uptake rate in counselled low-risk women may be as low as 40%. It is unlikely that differences of this magnitude could be accounted for by differences in the social and demographic mix of the populations served. In the present state of knowledge therefore, high uptake rates for serum screening for

Down's syndrome should not be interpreted as providing evidence of high acceptability. It is not clear that women understand the strengths or limitations of the screening being offered to them, and uptake rates seem to depend quite strongly on how the test is presented.

Having acknowledged that many women are making decisions about testing on the basis of incomplete information, it is also valid to investigate the decision-making process in circumstances of complete information and explicitly specified values. Decision analysis is a method for breaking complex problems down into manageable parts; all possible outcomes are identified, and probabilities (derived from the literature or from experience) are attached to them. An individual's values are then elicited for each of those outcomes, and 'utilities' calculated (the products of values and probabilities) for the various branches of the decision tree. The 'best' decision is the one which leads to the outcome with the highest utility, i.e. the decision which maximizes overall benefit. In a paper reviewing the application of decision analysis to obstetric care and prenatal diagnosis, Lilford and Thornton (1992) argue that although the full-blown technique is unlikely to be incorporated into the management of individual patients, construction of a basic decision tree can clarify any major trade-offs involved, and this will in itself help to make better decisions. As Tversky and Kahnemann (1974) pointed out many years ago, the human mind is prone to many 'faulty heuristics' when making decisions; research using decision analysis may indicate ways of counteracting known biases, and help guide pregnant mothers and caregivers in the future.

The psychological costs and benefits to women undergoing prenatal diagnosis and screening have also been investigated by Marteau and colleagues. An early finding was the increased distress and anxiety associated with receiving false positive results from MSAFP testing (Marteau, Kidd, Cook, et al., 1988b). Poor understanding of the test was considered an important contributory factor, particularly in younger women. A more recent report by the same team however found no evidence of an increase in anxiety on receipt of an abnormal alpha-fetoprotein result (Marteau, Kidd, Michie et al., 1993). Richards and Green (1993) speculate that the routine nature of MSAFP testing, and the lack of a numerical risk score when presenting results may lead to apparent indifference of this kind. When Marteau and colleagues looked at the psychological effects of amniocentesis, they found that tested women had significantly lower anxiety levels in the third trimester of pregnancy than women who had not been tested (Marteau, Johnston, Shaw et al., 1989b).

Serum testing for Down's syndrome has been introduced relatively recently. Comparable psychological data are not yet available, and recent debate has centered on the problems caused by inadequate counselling, reactions to positive results, and the issue of informed consent (Marteau, 1993; Statham and Green, 1993; BMJ correspondence, 1993). Roelofsen, Kamerbeek, Tymstra et al. (1993a) reported very positive attitudes to serum screening in their Dutch sample, but commented that many women seemed unaware of possible drawbacks. The same team reported (1993b) that positive triple test results did indeed lead to anxiety. Statham and Green (1993) reported considerable distress after screen positive results, with some anxieties continuing after negative amniocentesis results, or even after the birth of a healthy baby. All agreed that good information is likely to reduce the distress caused by unexpected test results.

All of this suggests that psychological reactions to prenatal testing are very sensitive to external factors. One factor which is potentially very influential is the nature of the technology used.

Ultrasound

By the mid 1980s the use of ultrasound during the second trimester had become a routine, and hence almost universal, part of antenatal care. Scans are used to determine how many babies there are, and to estimate their gestational age, as well as to look for fetal abnormalities. They are also used to gather information about the position of the placenta. Scans carried out at different gestational ages will perform some of these functions better than others. On the other hand, it is difficult to carry out any one function properly without also to some extent carrying out the others. Even if a mother is opposed to prenatal screening she may be scanned for other reasons, raising important issues of ethics and informed consent. It is in fact very unusual for formal consent to be sought for scanning; it is presented as an integral part of care which women have to be very well-informed and very assertive to resist.

Given its near universality, it might be assumed that the case for routine ultrasound scanning was well established. This is not in fact true. It is fully acknowledged that scans which are clinically indicated, perhaps because of suspicions about the baby's growth or lack of movement, provide information of immense value. Screen positive results on other tests, e.g. MSAFP, may also indicate the need for a scan if the mother wishes it. The question at issue is whether routine scanning of all pregnant women, i.e. including those with no clinical indications, improves perinatal outcomes. Put another way: does a routine scan pick up problems that are not detectable by other screening tests, or by clinical investigation? The RADIUS trial (Routine Antenatal Diagnostic Imaging with Ultrasound) randomized 15 151 low-risk pregnant women in the United States to either routine ultrasound at 15–22 weeks and again at 31–35 weeks, or to a control group given scans only for medical reasons identified by their doctors. The project team concluded, '... this practice-based trial demonstrates that among low risk pregnant women, ultrasound screening does not improve perinatal outcome. Potential benefits such as satisfying patients' desires for assurance that there are no fetal anomalies must be weighed against the unnecessary anxiety entailed in the examinations, and the risks of over-treatment due to false positive diagnoses. The adoption of routine ultrasound screening in the United States would add considerably to the cost of care in pregnancy, with no improvement in perinatal outcome' (Ewigman, Crane, Frigoletto et al., 1993). A report of another study, this time from Australia, showed a possible risk of one-third more cases of intrauterine growth retardation in a group randomized to receive five scans compared to a group receiving only one. The increase was statistically significant, but because of the number of statistical comparisons made in the study, the authors acknowledged that it might be a chance effect, rather than evidence of a cause and effect relationship. Their results however led them to conclude, 'Repeated prenatal ultrasound imaging ... should be restricted to those women to whom the information is likely to be of clinical benefit' (Newnham, Evans, Michael et al., 1993).

In response to these papers, a number of commentators have argued that the benefits of routine ultrasound are psychological: parents like to see their baby, and value the reassurance that a normal scan provides. They value it so much that many are willing to pay for a scan if their health care system does not provide one (Obstetrical and Gynecological Survey, 1994).

Justifications for clinical care

Similar arguments have been advanced regarding antenatal care in general. Women in Britain have an average of 15 antenatal checks during pregnancy. From a medical point of view, it is likely that no more than five are necessary, plus simple blood pressure checking in the last three months. One eminent professor of obstetrics and gynaecology has asked: 'Why then has such a pattern of largely ineffective ritual persisted in antenatal care?' (Steer, 1993). The explanation he inclines towards is again a psychological one: women are believed to like the present arrangements and find them reassuring. Steer also believes that doctors and midwives are afraid of missing something if they fail to conform to the expected pattern of care, which in Britain is essentially unchanged from that specified by Dame Janet Campbell in the 1920s. For all kinds of psychological and sometimes legal reasons, it seems to be very difficult to stop providing certain elements of care, even when effective justification for them is lacking. For doctors and midwives who have spent years delivering the old style of care, cognitive dissonance regarding the value of that time seems likely to contribute to their reluctance to change. Additionally, in the current political climate, NHS staff are quick to suspect that financial motives underlie apparently scientific decisions to change patterns of care. Such suspicions are very difficult to refute.

In both cases then – routine ultrasound and the traditional pattern of antenatal attendances – care which is of uncertain value clinically continues to be provided on the grounds that it is of value psychologically. No proper evaluations of psychological outcomes have however been conducted. It seems at least possible that the observed psychological value comes in large measure from the belief that one is receiving something of clinical value. If the latter was questioned, the former may evaporate, or at least diminish. This possibility has not been tested.

Attitudes to technology

It seems at least plausible that, even when adequately counselled, women's attitudes to screening tests may partly reflect their attitudes to the technology used. Rightly or wrongly, ultrasound carries very positive connotations for most women, and it may be particularly difficult for them to appreciate that this familiar and apparently benign technology can be used for the less benign purpose of screening for fetal abnormalities. Green, Snowdon and Statham (1993) provide vivid examples of apparent confusions, citing one case of a woman who was given an extra unexplained scan following her decision not to have MSAFP screening; but also describing women who were outraged at the suggestion that they should forgo scanning if they did not want other screening tests. It seems likely therefore, that even after counselling, uptake of Down's screening by ultrasound will be higher than uptake for serum testing. The data are not yet available to test this hypothesis. To take the argument one step further, it may also be that a women's interpretation of a particular risk figure is also coloured by her understanding of the technology used to calculate it: interpreting a picture may be seen as inherently more problematic than doing something with blood in a laboratory, or alternatively, it may seem more understandable, controllable and reliable than a number produced by a machine. On the other hand again, the demonstration of a physical change, visible on a scan, may be worrying to women in its own right, and not only as a marker for Down's syndrome. It may be difficult to exorcize this worry. The general idea that 'the medium may influence the message' has implications for screening programmes beyond the Down's screening example discussed here.

Because the technology has become available only recently, nothing is known about the psychological effects of earlier as opposed to later ultrasound scanning. Scanning in the second trimester arouses generally positive psychological responses, provided that adequate feedback is given (e.g. Tsoi and Hunter, 1987). There is however some evidence that when the purpose of anomaly scanning is made explicit, then positive attitudes are less likely to be found (Thorpe, Harker, Pike and Marlow, 1993).

Early claims that scanning increases bonding have not been substantiated, although it may bring it forward in time. Short-term effects on maternal health behaviours, such as smoking and visiting the dentist, have been shown in studies which gave mothers detailed feedback about the fetus during ultrasonography. This work has been reviewed by Lumley (1990).

Overall, scanning does not seem to reduce maternal anxiety. What seems to happen is that the process of scanning increases anxiety, then positive feedback reduces it again. After reviewing this literature, Lumley (1990) drew attention to 'slips and shadows: the diagnostic toxicity of prenatal ultrasound scans'. She argued that in everyday practice, feedback is not always of high quality; there may be 'slips of the tongue, incorrect diagnoses, identification of structures that cannot be deciphered, and language that is unfamiliar and alarming to mothers'. When abnormalities are detected, the effect on staff as well as parents can be profound (Ursing and Jorgensen, 1993). Support mechanisms for staff finding themselves in these circumstances are often insufficiently developed.

Paradox

It will by now be apparent that antenatal care in general, and prenatal testing in particular are founded on a paradox. Information and counselling before prenatal testing may help women cope with the news of an abnormal result; but a woman whose result proves to be normal probably experiences more anxiety as a result of being given information than she would have done without it. The overwhelming majority of women have pregnancies free of major problems, and go on to deliver normal babies. The challenge is how to balance the benefit to the few against the psychological cost – even a minor cost – to the many. Policies of ultrasound scanning and MSAFP testing for neural tube defects have succeeded in keeping most people happy by not being explicit about the purpose of the tests. Maintaining a service run along these lines is one thing, but introducing a new service run this way is something else. The arrival of serum screening for Down's syndrome has meant that attempts must be made to inform mothers adequately about prenatal testing, even if no-one knows at the moment how that should best be done, and even if resources for counselling have not increased in line with technological developments.

In a survey of obstetricians by Green (1994), nearly half the sample said they did not have adequate resources for counselling women offered serum screening for Down's; 88% reported that anxiety in women receiving false positive results was a problem for their screening service, and 81% thought that women's understanding of the test was a problem. Lack of knowledge amongst staff has been identified as a barrier to providing women with adequate information, and a staff training policy has been advocated (Marteau, Slack, Kidd and Shaw, 1992b; Smith, Slack, Shaw and Marteau, 1994; Smith, Shaw and Marteau, 1994). When it is appreciated that the great majority of pregnant women in the UK are now being offered serum screening, the scale of the problem becomes apparent.

The container and its contents

One distinction which should be made when giving women information about prenatal testing has been highlighted by Green and Statham (1993). The monitoring of maternal haemoglobin and blood pressure, for example, are 'tests to see whether the mother is a healthy container for her unborn child'. Importantly, if problems are detected, some corrective action can often be taken: iron tablets may be prescribed or rest advised. Tests of fetal well-being are tests of the contents rather than the container; and crucially, when abnormalities in the fetus are identified, it is very rare that anything positive can be done. Parents of a seriously damaged baby are usually faced with a single decision: whether or not to terminate the pregnancy.

Scans and blood tests provide information about container and contents. A reassuring justification often offered is that a test is being conducted 'to make sure that everything is alright' (McIntyre, 1987, cited in Green, Statham and Snowdon, 1992). This may be true when a sample of blood is used to measure the mother's haemoglobin, for example; but if the same blood sample is also used to test for Down's syndrome, then the implications of that reassuring phrase can be seriously misleading.

Carrier screening

The antenatal clinic can be a very confusing place in which women are bombarded with information. They are likely to be counselled about their diet and about smoking, and to have discussions about preparing for the birth itself and about parentcraft, all in addition to undergoing various tests of their own physical well-being and receiving information about prenatal screening. The list is not finished however, because increasingly women attending for antenatal care are also being targeted for other kinds of genetic screening, e.g. carrier detection for cystic fibrosis (CF). This is an autosomal recessive disease with an incidence of about 1 in 2 500 births. Figures suggest that in the general population of

10 000 people, 400 will be a carrier of cystic fibrosis, but only 16 will have a partner who is also a carrier. Although in principle carrier detection can be carried out at any age, pilot screening programmes have, to date, concentrated on adults of child-bearing age, and on those already pregnant. Screening will detect approximately 65% of couples where both parents are carriers. In these circumstances, each of their children has a 1 in 4 risk of suffering from cystic fibrosis. If the woman is already pregnant, this information can be used to guide decisions about invasive prenatal diagnostic testing and the possibility of abortion.

Reviewing studies of the uptake of pregnancy screening for cystic fibrosis, Raeburn (1994) noted that 'if an offer was made directly by an interested health professional the take up rate exceeded 70%'. In non-pregnant groups the figures are much lower, and taken together with other work suggest that people are not actively opposed to being tested but are not actively interested in being tested either. Richards and Green (1993) argue that interest is low because most people have not encountered CF and do not have anxieties that their children may have the disease. Further, lay beliefs about inheritance may falsely lead people to conclude that if they are healthy, then it is impossible for them to pass on a genetic disease. Such individuals would accept testing only in a situation where it was easier to accept than to refuse.

A study of the psychological consequences of carrier screening for cystic fibrosis in the antenatal clinic (Mennie, Gilfillan, Compton et al., 1992; Mennie, Compton, Gilfillan et al., 1993) found that stress was of short duration: it increased in women identified as carriers, but decreased again when the partner was found not to carry a detectable CF allele. The authors concluded that the main resource implication of their programme was in providing counselling support for carrier women during that period. Studies of CF carrier testing in non-pregnant populations have suggested that residual anxiety may persist (Watson, Mayall, Lamb et al., 1992); and again the role of counselling has been emphasized. Another study has identified false reassurance (i.e. people thinking they were less at risk than they actually were) as more of a problem than persistent anxiety (Bekker, Denniss, Modell et al., 1994). These authors point out that little is known about how well people remember information on carrier status, or about whether that information influences their future reproductive decisions.

Conclusion

Drawing a number of threads together, it becomes clear that the provision of information and psychological support to women facing prenatal testing is inadequate. New procedures are introduced with little regard paid to how they will be perceived by women, either on their own, or as part of an overall package of antenatal care. Counselling would seem to be of particular importance in circumstances where women are being offered more than one sort of test. The possibilities for confusion, for example, between Down's and CF testing, are apparent and have potentially very serious implications.

As Richards amongst others has pointed out (1989), 'There are too many examples in the history of medicine of technological research and development running far ahead of our knowledge of how to use and deploy what is available.'

In an earlier review of the quality of controlled clinical trials of ultrasound in obstetrics, Thacker (1985) wrote, 'Finally, it is not enough to determine that a screening procedure is efficacious, the human and monetary costs of the procedure must also be assessed, and the effectiveness, safety and acceptability of subsequent interventions must be considered.' It has to be acknowledged that, to date, such counsel has had relatively little effect on the development and introduction of the technology of prenatal screening.

Applications

1. Understanding of risk

Most people find the ideas of probability and of risk difficult to understand, and time and skill are required to give parents all the information they need to make informed choices about prenatal testing. Resources for counselling and support need to be provided when prenatal screening programmes are offered.

2. False positive test results

Screen positive test results can produce high levels of anxiety that may persist even after the baby has been found to be normal. Good information is thought to be particularly important in alleviating the distress caused by results of this kind.

3. Confusions

When new tests are introduced (e.g. carrier screening for cystic fibrosis) or new applications found for familiar technologies (e.g. ultrasound screening for Down's syndrome), the possibilities for confusion increase. Special efforts should be made in these circumstances to ensure that parents understand the purpose of each test and can make a genuine decision about whether they wish to have it or not.

Further reading

Abramsky, L. and Chapple, J. (eds) (1993). *The human side of prenatal diagnosis*. London: Chapman and Hall.

Green, J. and Richards, M. (eds) (1993). Psychological aspects of fetal screening and the new genetics. Special issue, *Journal of Reproductive and Infant Psychology*, **11**, 1.

Green, J. and Statham, H. (1993). Testing for fetal abnormality in routine antenatal care. *Midwifery*, **9**, 124–35.

References

Bekker, H., Denniss, G., Modell, M., Bobrow, M. and Marteau, T. M. (1994). The impact of population based screening for carriers of cystic fibrosis. *Journal of Medical Genetics*, **31**, 364–8.

BMJ correspondence, Serum screening for Down's syndrome. *British Medical Journal*, **307**, 500–2.

Ewigman, B., Crane, J., Frigoletto, F. et al. (1993). Effect of prenatal ultrasound screening on perinatal outcome. *New England Journal of Medicine*, **329**, 821–7.

Faden, R. R., Chwalow, A. J., Orel-Crosby, E., Holtzman, N. A., Chase, G. A. and Leonard, C. O. (1985). What participants understand about a maternal serum alpha-fetoprotein screening programme. *American Journal of Public Health*, **75**, 1381–4.

Green, J. (1994). Serum screening for Down's syndrome: experiences of obstetricians in England and Wales. *British Medical Journal*, **309**, 769–72.

Green, J., Statham, H. and Snowdon, C. (1992). Screening for fetal abnormalities: attitudes and experiences. In *Obstetrics in the 1990s: current controversies* (T. Chard and M. P. M. Richards, eds). London: MacKeith Press.

Green, J., Snowdon, C. and Statham, H. (1993). Pregnant women's attitudes to abortion and prenatal screening. *Journal of Reproductive and Infant Psychology*, **11**, 31–9.

Green, J. and Statham, H. (1993). Testing for fetal abnormality in routine antenatal care. *Midwifery*, **9**, 124–35.

Johnston, M. and Marteau, T. M. (1990). Psychological aspects of prenatal screening. *Medical Research Council News*, **47**, 8–9.

Lilford, R. J. and Thornton, J. G. (1992). Making difficult decisions. In *Obstetrics in the 1990s: current controversies* (T. Chard and M. P. M. Richards, eds). London: MacKeith Press.

Lumley, J. (1990). Through a glass darkly: ultrasound and prenatal bonding. *Birth*, **17**, 214–17.

Marteau, T. M. (1993). Psychological consequences of screening for Down's syndrome. *British Medical Journal*, **307**, 146–7.

Marteau, T. M., Johnston, M., Plenicar, M., Shaw, R. W. and Slack, J. (1988a). Development of a self-administered questionnaire to measure women's knowledge of prenatal screening and diagnostic tests. *Journal of Psychosomatic Research*, **32**, 403–8.

Marteau, T. M., Kidd, J., Cook, R., Johnston, M., Michie, S., Shaw, R. W. and Slack, J. (1988b). Screening for Down's syndrome (letter). *British Medical Journal*, **297**, 1469.

Marteau, T. M., Johnston, M., Shaw, R. W. and Slack, J. (1989a). Factors influencing the uptake of screening for open neural-tube defects and amniocentesis to test for Down's syndrome. *British Journal of Obstetrics and Gynaecology*, **96**, 739–48.

Marteau, T. M., Johnston, M., Shaw, R. W., Michie, S., Kidd, J. and New, M. (1989b). The impact of prenatal screening and diagnostic testing upon the cognitions, emotions and behaviour of pregnant women. *Journal of Psychosomatic Research*, **33**, 7–16.

Marteau, T. M., Kidd, J. and Cook, R. (1991). Perceived risk not actual risk predicts uptake of amniocentesis. *British Journal of Obstetrics and Gynaecology*, **98**, 282–6.

Marteau, T. M., Johnston, M., Kidd, J., Michie, S. and Cook, R. (1992a). Psychological models in predicting uptake of prenatal screening. *Psychology and Health*, **6**, 13–22.

Marteau, T. M., Slack, J., Kidd, J. and Shaw, R. W. (1992b). Presenting a routine screening test in antenatal care: practice observed. *Public Health*, **106**, 131–41.

Marteau, T. M., Kidd, J., Michie, S., Cook, R., Johnston, M. and Shaw, R. W. (1993). Anxiety, knowledge and satisfaction in women receiving false positive results on routine prenatal testing: a randomized controlled trial. *Journal of Psychosomatic Obstetrics and Gynaecology*, **14**, 185–96.

Mennie, M. E., Gilfillan, A., Compton, M et al. (1992). Prenatal screening for cystic fibrosis. *Lancet*, **340**, 214–16.

Mennie, M. E., Compton, M., Gilfillan, A. et al. (1993). Prenatal screening for cystic fibrosis: psychological effects on carriers and their partners. *Journal of Medical Genetics*, **30**, 543–8.

Newnham, J. P., Evans, S. F., Michael, C. A., Stanley, F. J. and Landau, L. I. (1993). Effects of frequent ultrasound during pregnancy: a randomised controlled trial. *Lancet*, **342**, 887–91.

Nicolaides, K. H., Azar, G., Byrne, D., Mansur, C. and Marks, K. (1992). Fetal nuchal translucency: Ultrasound screening for chromosomal defects in the first trimester of pregnancy. *British Medical Journal*, **304**, 867–9.

Obstetrical and Gynecological Survey (1994). Review of paper by Ewigman et al., **49**, 86–9.

Raeburn, J. A. (1994). Screening for carriers of cystic fibrosis. *British Medical Journal*, **308**, 1451–2.

Reynolds, T. M., Nix, A. B., Dunstan, F. D. and Dawson, A. J. (1993). Age specific detection and false positive rates: an aid to counselling in Down's Syndrome risk screening. *Obstetrics and Gynaecology*, **81**, 447–50.

Richards, M. P. M. (1989). Social and ethical problems of fetal diagnosis and screening. *Journal of Reproductive and Infant Psychology*, **7**, 171–85.

Richards, M. P. M. and Green, J. M. (1993). Attitudes toward prenatal screening for fetal abnormality and detection of carriers of genetic disease: a discussion paper. *Journal of Reproductive and Infant Psychology*, **11**, 49–56.

Roelofsen, E. E. C., Kamerbeek, L. I., Tymstra, T. J., Beekhuis, J. R. and Mantingh, A. (1993a). Women's opinions on the offer and use of maternal serum screening. *Prenatal Diagnosis*, **13**, 741–7.

Roelofsen, E. E. C., Kamerbeek, L. I. and Tymstra, T. (1993b). Chances and choices. Psycho-social consequences of maternal serum screening. A report from the Netherlands. *Journal of Reproductive and Infant Psychology*, **11**, 41–7.

Schulte-Vallentin, M. and Schindler, H. (1992). Non-echogenic nuchal oedema as a marker in trisomy 21 screening. *Lancet*, **339**, 1053.

Seror, V., Muller, F., Moatti, J. P., Le Gales, C. and Boue, A. (1993). Economic assessment of maternal serum screening for Down's syndrome using human chorionic gonadotrophin. *Prenatal Diagnosis*, **13**, 281–92.

Sheldon, T. and Simpson, J. (1991). Appraisal of a new scheme for prenatal screening of Down's syndrome. *British Medical Journal*, **302**, 1133–6.

Shiloh, S. and Saxe, L. (1989). Perception of risk in genetic counselling. *Psychology and Health*, **3**, 45–61.

Smith, D. K., Shaw, R. W. and Marteau, T. M. (1994). Informed consent to undergo serum screening for Down's syndrome: the gap between policy and practice. *British Medical Journal*, **309**, 776.

Smith, D. K., Slack, J., Shaw, R. W. and Marteau, T. M. (1994). Lack of knowledge in health professionals: a barrier to providing information to patients? *Quality in Health Care*, **3**, 75–8.

Statham, H. and Green, J. (1993). Serum screening for Down's syndrome: some women's experiences. *British Medical Journal*, **307**, 174–6.

Steer, P. (1993). Rituals in antenatal care – do we need them? *British Medical Journal*, **307**, 697.

Thacker, S. B. (1985). Quality of controlled clinical trials. The case of imaging ultrasound in obstetrics: a review. *British Journal of Obstetrics and Gynaecology*, **92**, 437–44.

Thornton, J., Hewson, J., Lilford, R. J. et al. (1995). A randomised trial of three methods of giving information about prenatal testing. *British Medical Journal*, **311**, 1127–30.

Thorpe, K., Harker, L., Pike, A. and Marlow, N. (1993). Women's views of ultrasonography; A comparison of women's experiences of antenatal ultrasound screening with cerebral ultrasound of their newborn infant. *Social Science and Medicine*, **36**, 3, 311–15.

Tsoi, M. M. and Hunter, M. (1987). Ultrasound scanning in pregnancy: consumer reactions. *Journal of Reproductive and Infant Psychology*, **5**, 43–8.

Tversky, A. and Kahnemann, D. (1974). Judgement under uncertainty: heuristics and biases. *Science*, **185**, 1124–31.

Tymstra, T. (1989). The imperative character of medical technology and the meaning of anticipated decision regret. *International Journal of Technology Assessment in Health Care*, **5**, 207–13.

Ursing, J. and Jorgensen, C. (1993). Ultrasound screening during pregnancy: psychological strain experienced by the investigating staff. *Ultrasound in Obstetrics and Gynaecology*, **3**, 100. (Extract reprinted in *Obstetrical and Gynaecological Survey 1994*, **49**, 11–13.)

Wald, N., Cuckle, H. S., Densem, J. W. et al. (1988). Maternal serum screening for Down's syndrome in early pregnancy. *British Medical Journal*, **297**, 883–7.

Wald, N., Kennard, A., Densem, J., Cuckle, H. S., Chard, T. and Butler, L. (1992). Antenatal maternal serum screening for Down's syndrome: results of a demonstration project. *British Medical Journal*, **305**, 391–4.

Watson, E. K., Mayall, E. S., Lamb, J., Chapple, J. and Williamson, R. (1992). Psychological and social consequences of community carrier screening programme for cystic fibrosis. *Lancet*, **340**, 217–20.

7

Miscarriage

Rosanne Cecil and Pauline Slade

It is seldom realized that miscarriage is a much more common consequence of conception than birth. As Rosanne Cecil and Pauline Slade discuss in this chapter, this life event often occurs without the knowledge of the couple involved and even when it is known about, is frequently hidden from the wider society. However, substantial research has been carried out into its psychological consequences and the authors have been innovative in relating this to a variety of theoretical perspectives.

As the dividing lines between miscarriage and stillbirth are difficult to draw, this chapter should be read in conjunction with Chapter 12. The first volume of the series also contains a related chapter on abortion.

... a death before a birth is itself the ultimate paradox. We are at one moment nurturing life and the next minute embracing death ...

(Hey, 1989)

What is miscarriage?

Miscarriage, also known as spontaneous abortion, is defined in the United Kingdom as the involuntary loss of the fetus from the womb prior to the legal age of viability of 24 weeks. Around one in five clinically recognized pregnancies end in miscarriage. Early embryonic loss may be a great deal higher; it has been estimated that 75% of all conceptions end in fetal death, the majority of these occurring without the knowledge of the woman. It can thus be seen that the dividing line between infertility and pregnancy loss at a very early stage of development is a rather hazy one. At the other end of the process of pregnancy the distinction between a late miscarriage and a stillbirth is similarly a matter of changing definitions; until recently a miscarriage was defined as the loss of a fetus prior to 28 weeks' gestation.

Causes of miscarriage

There are a number of different causes of miscarriage. The most common reason for a miscarriage to occur is that the chromosomes of the fetus are abnormal in one of a number of ways. The incidence of chromosomal abnormalities in abortuses is around 50%; this compares with a rate of around 5% in stillborn infants and 0.5% in liveborn infants (Simpson and Bombard, 1987). Some anomalies have been observed only amongst abortuses (Kline and Stein, 1987). These anomalies are thus incompatible with life. It is this which lies behind the oft-repeated well-meaning but uncomforting phrase, 'it is nature's way' (i.e. of preventing the birth of a severely sick and malformed child) familiar to so many women who have miscarried.

In many cases, however, chromosomally normal fetuses are miscarried. There are a number of reasons why this might occur. Infections of one kind or another pose a risk to a pregnancy. Certain viruses are known to cause the baby to develop abnormally and thus to be at risk of miscarriage. The best known of these is German measles (rubella). Other viral infections such as chickenpox, measles, mumps and influenza may cause a miscarriage if contracted during the early months of pregnancy.

Bacterial infections in animals such as brucellosis and chlamydia may cause miscarriage in women who are in contact with farm animals. Listeria is another bacterial infection which has been associated with miscarriage. Indeed a great many infectious agents are suspected of having a causal role in pregnancy loss. Charles and Larsen (1987) suggest that it may be the case that any infection which results in septicaemia can result in a miscarriage.

Other factors which have been implicated in miscarriage are uterine abnormalities, multiple pregnancies, certain medical conditions such as uncontrolled diabetes or thyroid dysfunction, certain medical procedures, immunological factors and environmental factors.

The likelihood of any one pregnancy ending in miscarriage is dependent on a number of different factors. Regan, Braude and Trembath (1989) suggest that past reproductive history may be the most relevant predictive factor in the outcome of a subsequent pregnancy. They found that the miscarriage rate was significantly higher amongst multigravidas (14%) than among primagravidas (5%). Women whose last pregnancy had been successful had a miscarriage rate of 5% whereas women whose last pregnancy had ended in miscarriage had a miscarriage rate of 20%. Maternal age is also a factor in the risk of miscarriage; there is an increased incidence of miscarriage beyond the age of 35.

Following a miscarriage most women go on to have a successful pregnancy. A proportion of women, however, have three or more miscarriages consecutively. Recurrent miscarriage, as this is called, is more likely to be due to factors other than chromosomal abnormalities. According to Warburton and Strobino (1987) the most common group of recurrent aborters are those who, often relatively late in gestation, abort chromosomally normal conceptions.

The management of miscarriage

The management of miscarriage can be considered as falling into two areas: the immediate management of a woman presenting with a miscarriage and the management of a woman who has had recurrent miscarriages.

The immediate management of a woman who presents with an incomplete and inevitable miscarriage is to minimize blood loss and the risk of infection. The majority of women who miscarry are seen in hospital where it is likely that the procedure of surgical curettage, to remove the products of conception, will be undertaken. Unless there are complications, women will usually spend only a short time in hospital (around 24 hours) before they are discharged.

While policy differs from hospital to hospital it is generally the case that unless a woman miscarries on three or more (sometimes two or more) occasions, investigations will not be undertaken as to the cause of miscarriage. Thus a woman who has had no more than one or two miscarriages is unlikely to be offered any form of treatment. One or two miscarriages are generally considered to be due to random factors. More than two miscarriages suggest that a specific cause may be to blame. In the case of women who miscarry repeatedly a number of tests may be undertaken in an attempt to determine the possible cause or causes. Which tests are offered may vary from clinician to clinician. Nevertheless it is likely that blood samples, from both the woman and her partner, will be taken and a hysterosalpingogram carried out in order to check for any uterine abnormalities. In addition thyroid function tests and screening for auto-immune disease may be undertaken.

Women's experiences of miscarriage

A number of books which have been written primarily for women who have suffered a miscarriage, such as those by Oakley, McPherson and Roberts (1984), Leroy (1988), Hey, Itzin, Saunders and Speakman (1989) and Moulder (1990) present, by way of women's personal accounts, a very vivid picture of some women's experiences of miscarriage. Recent psychological and sociological studies have attempted to focus on certain aspects of women's experiences and coping behaviour in an attempt to understand those factors which have a positive and those which have a negative impact upon women. Researchers have looked, for example, at hospital care (Helstrom and Victor, 1987; Jackman, McGee and Turner, 1991; Moohan, Ashe and Cecil, 1994) and general practitioner care (Friedman, 1989; Roberts, 1991); and have conducted follow-up studies involving different timescales including studies of women during and after subsequent pregnancies (Cordle and Prettyman, 1994; Statham and Green, 1994). Such studies are discussed in some detail later in this chapter.

Hospital care

Studies into hospital care have highlighted a number of areas of concern to women including the appropriateness of the accommodation provided in hospitals (women are variously accommodated in gynaecological wards, antenatal or postnatal wards; single rooms or open wards); issues of privacy; the sensitive question of the management of the baby's remains; the attitudes of staff and, perhaps most important of all, the issue of explanations and information-giving.

The manner in which information and explanations are given and the way in which hospital procedures are carried out may have an impact upon a woman's immediate and long-term sense of well-being (Kaplan, Greenfield and Ware, 1989; Carel, Blondel, Lelong et al., 1992). As miscarriage is a very common event and normally only requires routine medical and nursing care, hospital staff may not appreciate the significance a miscarriage may have for a woman and her partner. Information which is given at this time needs to be conveyed clearly and sensitively. Many women who have had a miscarriage have a great desire and need for information about their own miscarriage and about mis-carriage in general.

The need for information and explanations continues, for many, after hospital discharge. A number of studies have indicated the importance of some kind of follow-up, either at the hospital or with the woman's own GP (Hamilton, 1989;

Jackman, McGee and Turner, 1991). Some hospitals and health authorities provide information leaflets or booklets for women. Although generally welcomed by women who have miscarried, the specific impact of such literature has yet to be evaluated.

Hospital procedures may be experienced as neutral, alternatively they may increase or lessen feelings of distress. It is, as yet, unclear whether the widespread use of the ultrasound scan, by which a woman can see an image of the fetus at an increasingly early stage of gestation, helps or hinders her in coming to terms with miscarriage if the pregnancy should subsequently be lost. While Layne (1992) writes that 'sonogram images facilitate the perception of the fetus as a separate individual, even before quickening' and 'it is self-evident that the greater the feelings of involvement, attachment, love for a desired child, the greater the potential sense of loss', she goes on to note that the impact of sonogram images on those whose pregnancies end without a live birth has largely been ignored.

The very language which is used within the hospital setting may cause distress to a woman. Connolly (1989) and Chalmers (1992) discuss those terms commonly used by medical and nursing staff which may have negative connotations for women such as 'failed pregnancy' and 'incompetent cervix'. Chalmers suggests that although these terms may have objective medical meanings for doctors, for women, focusing on the words 'failed' and 'incompetent' their meaning may be very different. Oakley, McPherson and Roberts (1984) among others, have written of the distress which the use of the term 'abortion' as opposed to 'miscarriage' may cause to women. Roberts (1989) discusses how the use of differing terminology for what is lost, 'a baby' or 'the products of conception', is a reflection of the differing perspectives of women who have miscarried and of health professionals.

Health professionals and pregnancy loss

In her study of staff at four London hospitals and 22 women who had either had a late miscarriage, a stillbirth or a perinatal loss, Lovell (1983) found that health workers shared an assumption of 'hierarchies of sadness'. That is, health workers considered that 'the earlier the pregnancy failed, the "lesser" the loss, making miscarriages less sad than stillbirth; and stillbirth less sad than losing a baby who had lived'. Lovell's study, however, challenged such an assumption. She found that the mothers of babies who had briefly lived after birth seemed able to make better sense of their loss. They were better able to mourn; their baby's existence, although so short, had been acknowledged and the loss therefore recognized as being of considerable significance.

Friedman (1989) interviewed 67 women four weeks after they left hospital following a miscarriage. Eighty-eight per cent of the women had contacted their GP prior to hospital admission. They were asked about both the care and the information which they had received from their GP. While most women were at least moderately satisfied with the levels of care which they received, there was a certain amount of dissatisfaction. The major reason for this was the 'mismatch between the patients' and the doctors' perceptions of patients' needs'. The women and the GPs held different perceptions of the seriousness and the importance of the miscarriage or threatened miscarriage. With echoes of Lovell (1983), Friedman (1989) notes that 'Emotionally the experience of early miscarriage may be as distressing as that of late miscarriage or a stillbirth but it is not recognized as such and is therefore a more unshared problem that the other two losses'.

Marking the event

A number of writers have made the observation that there are no culturally shared rituals and practices which mark the loss of a pregnancy before term. Chalmers (1992) suggests that:

> The lack of recognition of the loss as a baby, particularly if the miscarriage takes place in very early pregnancy; the absence of any burial ceremony to mark the recognition of lost life; the inability to identify a place of remembrance such as a burial site; the lack of social recognition of the woman as a mother even if only of a baby that has died, and the expectation that mourning is not needed or is inappropriate in the event of early pregnancy loss, may make mourning more difficult.

That is, miscarriage lacks what anthropologists refer to as 'rites de passage' (following Van Gennep, 1909). The significance of the loss of the pregnancy is rarely acknowledged by any one other than the would-be mother and, in many cases, her partner and close family. In response to this, some pregnancy loss support groups have begun to create their own rituals of mourning and remembrance (see Layne (1990) on such groups in the USA). The manner in which the remains of the baby/fetus/products of conception are dealt with is central to this issue. Kohner (1992) in a study conducted for the Stillbirth and Neonatal Death Society (SANDS) observed that, 'respectful procedures for the disposal of the bodies of pre-viable babies tend to arise out of the acceptance of some fundamental ideas concerning the status of the baby's body or remains and the needs, if not also the rights, of the parents'. As miscarriage can occur at any stage during a pregnancy up until the 24th week of gestation (at which point the loss would be termed a stillbirth in the United Kingdom), what is lost, and what therefore needs disposal, may vary considerably. It may be 'a well formed baby, a body which was never well formed or which has partially or wholly disintegrated, a very tiny fetus, parts of a baby or fetus, or blood, tissue etc. which may or may not include identifiable parts' (Kohner, 1992). The needs and wishes of the parents may differ not only in terms of the nature of the pregnancy loss but also in terms of other factors such as religious and cultural identity and emotional and personal preferences. A survey of district health authorities (and their equivalent) throughout the United Kingdom revealed a wide variation in disposal procedures. While a few hospitals provided cremation or burial for all identifiable bodies, regardless of gestational age, elsewhere the bodies of pre-viable babies were incinerated with other hospital waste or disposed of via a waste disposal unit (Kohner, 1992). The work of SANDS, especially its publication offering guidelines for professionals in the field of miscarriage, stillbirth and neonatal death (SANDS, 1991), has done much to bring about changes in hospital policy and practice.

Psychological consequences of miscarriage

Women may vary considerably in their response to miscarriage. The emotional reactions to a miscarriage may range from outright relief and happiness to profound and serious psychopathology (Graves, 1987). However, it is only relatively recently that there have been systematic attempts to assess the psychological impact of miscarriage. If appropriate psychological care is to be provided then it is important to understand how women respond emotionally to this experience and to try to identify factors which may have predictive power. These issues are reviewed in greater detail by Slade (1994).

Information from several studies conducted in locations in Western Europe and North America suggests that there is probably some increased risk of significant depressive symptoms within the first month after a miscarriage with between one-fifth and a half of women affected in this way (Friedman and Gath, 1989; Carel, Blondel, Lelong et al., 1992; Prettyman, Cordle and Cook, 1993; Neugebauer, Kline, O'Connor et al., 1992). Many women also report considerable anxiety symptoms although the particular focus of their concerns has not been explored and remains unclear (Prettyman, Cordle and Cook, 1993; Tharpar and Tharpar, 1992; Cecil and Leslie, 1993). The effect of the passage of time on these feelings is still controversial with Prettyman, Cordle and Cook (1993) suggesting some resolution by three months after miscarriage for many with depressive symptoms. However this is contradicted by others (Garel, Blondel, Lelong et al., 1992; Neugebauer, Kline, O'Connor et al., 1992). Indeed Robinson, Stirtzinger, Stewart and Ralevski (1994) suggest that the seeming resolution at six months may be followed by an increase in depressive symptoms at one year which may possibly be construed as an anniversary effect. The temporal patterning for anxiety symptoms may also be complex. It appears that these may emerge at different times after the miscarriage, possibly with different foci for different individuals. For example, initial anxiety may concern the trauma of pain and bleeding whilst later anxiety may relate to implications for future pregnancies. In addition, low anxiety when it occurs initially may not be maintained. Cordle and Prettyman (1994) completed one of the longest follow-ups available at two years post miscarriage. Whilst neither anxiety or depression symptoms were elevated, one-quarter of women still thought about their miscarriage often or very often and two-thirds were at least moderately upset by these thoughts. As 12% reported thinking about this event often and being extremely distressed, as many as one in eight women could still be considered to be experiencing negative consequences. As noted earlier, Statham and Green (1994) found that women who had experienced a miscarriage are likely to show higher anxiety levels during a subsequent pregnancy than other pregnant women, and not unexpectedly they show a greater concern about miscarriage. However concern is diminished if a successful pregnancy has been experienced since the miscarriage.

Most research has focused upon the experiences of the woman herself. However, her partner's reactions are also important together with the effects of the event on their relationship. Robinson, Stirtzinger, Stewart and Ralevski (1994) assessed the quality of the marital relationship at points up to a year following miscarriage; the findings did not suggest any significant impact over time. However this area has received little investigation.

Factors which may help in predicting individual psychological distress

Understanding who is most at risk from negative emotional responses may elucidate the mechanisms that may be involved. A variety of factors have been considered and can be grouped according to five categories.

1. Demographic characteristics such as age, marital status, social class and parity.
2. General life history factors such as psychiatric history or bereavements.
3. Aspects of reproductive history such as infertility, therapeutic abortion or previous miscarriage.
4. Variables relating to the pregnancy such as gestational age and whether the pregnancy was planned.
5. Aspects of the process of miscarriage, degree of blood and/or pain, the stress of hospitalization and the nature of the care provided.

Demographic factors such as age, marital status, parity and social class do not appear to be consistent predictors of emotional responses (Friedman and Gath, 1989; Prettyman, Cordle and Cook, 1993; Tharpar and Tharpar, 1992). When considering general life history factors, the one repeated finding seems to be that individuals who have suffered significant psychological distress in the past are particularly vulnerable (Friedman and Gath, 1989; Prettyman, Cordle and Cook, 1993). The impact of previous infertility and particularly previous miscarriage is unclear with some authors suggesting increased negative emotional symptoms and others no such effect (Friedman and Gath, 1989; Garel, Blondel, Lelong et al., 1992; Jackman, McGee and Turner, 1991). These equivocal findings may be explained by the fact that such historical factors may be incorporated into the experience of miscarriage in different way. While for many, such histories may enhance the sense of loss, some women with previous infertility may respond less negatively because the process is viewed in terms of affirming their ability to become pregnant. Similarly, some women may habituate to the experience in the case of repeated miscarriage or, as the finding by Conway (1992) implies, there may be improved communication and support between partners. Variables defined in this sort of way may be poor predictors because they fail to relate consistently to individual's perceptions of the event.

Neither the duration of gestation nor the presence or absence of planning of the pregnancy seem to act as significant predictors of distress (Friedman and Gath, 1989; Prettyman, Cordle and Cook, 1993). Indeed whether the pregnancy was planned appears to yield contradictory results. Although it might be expected that women who had planned their pregnancies might be more adversely affected emotionally by the loss, this does not seem to be the case. Responses to the loss of an unplanned pregnancy may be complex. Some women may feel a sense of relief but this may be accompanied by feelings of guilt about not having wanted the pregnancy. In their paper concerning grieving characteristics following miscarriage, Leppert and Pahlka (1984) identified guilt as the strongest and the most difficult response to resolve and this may explain why whether a pregnancy was planned is a poor predictor. Again this emphasizes the fact that a woman's own ideas about the meaning of the event to her are likely to be important.

The final set of potential predictors focusing upon the actual experience of the miscarriage process, including the nature of hospital and follow-up experience have received relatively little systematic attention. However, there are tentative suggestions that aspects of care and follow-up may be relevant to subsequent emotional responses. Slade and Wills (1993) showed strong associations between symptoms of depression and anxiety three to four months post miscarriage and low satisfaction with hospital care. However such correlational associations must be treated with caution as it is known that current mood may influence memory (Teasdale and Barnard, 1993). There are also suggestions that a detailed telephone interview about the experience of miscarriage shortly after that event may have led to lower levels of depressive symptoms at six months in a study by Neugebauer, Kline, O'Connor et al. (1992).

In summary, the predictive value of the variables typically investigated is disappointing and one potential explanation for their lack of power is that they fail to access the meaning of the event to the individual. This highlights the inappropriate nature of many of the staff assumptions about which women will be most distressed (Lovell, 1983).

Models for understanding the experience of miscarriage

In attempting to assess the psychological effects of miscarriage many studies have made an implicit assumption that focusing upon bereavement, and, in particular, loss, is an appropriate way of understanding the experience of miscarriage. The implications are that an individual may be expected to progress through stages of disbelief, anger, yearning and resolution. An additional assumption is that the grief process and ultimate adaptation is facilitated by 'working through' (that is, expressing) feelings and confronting the loss (Graves, 1987). In bereavement research, workers are questioning the validity of the concept of stages and indeed even the idea that 'working through' is an essential component of positive adjustment in normal grief (Stroebe, 1992–93). After a major bereavement people are typically faced with many changes and the mechanisms underpinning an increase in depressive symptoms or increased mortality in those bereaved may extend beyond the experience of loss. Old social roles are relinquished and new ones must be embraced. In addition many new demands are made upon recently bereaved individuals as they must often take on responsibilities previously carried out by the person who has died. Many of these issues have a lesser relevance in the case of miscarriage and this experience does involve certain specific attributes which differ from other bereavements. For example in miscarriage the loss is of a baby who has not experienced a separate and independent existence. The woman has no specific memories of that person. She does not have to take on new responsibilities but anticipated new roles must be relinquished. However, she still loses the role of 'pregnant woman'. Loss in miscarriage therefore has some common characteristics and some differences to other bereavements. Understanding the emotional consequences of miscarriage only in terms of loss negates other potentially important aspects of the experience. Other models may contribute to our understanding of these issues.

During a miscarriage, women have often undergone considerable pain and loss of blood, been admitted to hospital and experienced a first ever operation under general anaesthetic. Such components are characteristic of what may be considered as traumatic events which often lead to symptoms of anxiety and intrusive experiences such as nightmares, flashbacks or unwanted memories of the event (Horowitz, 1975). There is certainly evidence, as already noted, that anxiety levels tend to be high after miscarriage. Some of the consequences of miscarriage, in terms of anxiety, can be understood as responses to a traumatic event. It may therefore be important to consider the process of experiencing miscarriage itself as a stressor. Slade and Lee (1995) found that one week after miscarriage women were experiencing such intrusive experiences with a frequency common in patients suffering from post-traumatic stress disorder. It seems likely that some of the emotional responses may be influenced by the process of the experience of miscarriage and not primarily the loss of the baby.

In addition, how people think about different experiences appears to be important in their emotional responses. For example, Lazarus and Folkman (1984) suggest that stress responses may occur when an appraisal of the demands of the situation suggests that these exceed the person's perceptions of their available coping resources. Women's views on the personal meaning of the experience are therefore likely to be important. It is clear that there is a need for the development of a theoretical model with the utility for understanding the experience and consequences of miscarriage and which has the capacity to incorporate elements reflecting the potentially traumatic aspects of the event stress responses and loss. Within this it is important to take into account the personal meaning of the event and hence the role of cognitive factors.

As theoretical understanding of emotional states has developed, the aetiological roles of thoughts or cognitions in emotional responses has been recognized. Cognitive theories of emotion essentially assume that events themselves do not cause distress but an individual's construction of those events and their concomitant thoughts will determine the emotional consequences (Scherer, 1984). While there is still debate about the directionality of the relationship between cognitions and emotions (Williams, Watts, Macleod and Matthews, 1988) such factors are clearly worthy of investigation in relation to miscarriage.

Cognitions about miscarriage may be influenced by many factors including characteristics of the individual and the experience and may be affected by input from others during and after the event. Robinson, Stirtzinger, Stewart and Ralevski (1994) suggest that there is an association between self blame and blame from others and subsequent depressive symptoms. Madden (1988) considered beliefs about causes of miscarriage and suggested that blame of the partner and a view that one had some control over the outcome of subsequent pregnancy were both associated with reports of feelings of depression. While there were few details about the representativeness of their sample, these findings were interesting as research in depression in general has suggested that feelings of helplessness or hopelessness rather than perceptions of control act as predictors (Abramson, Metalsky and Alloy, 1989). Tunaley, Slade and Duncan (1993) studied a small sample of women who had miscarried and considered how their beliefs related to their adaptation. An interesting innovation in this study was the inclusion of an assessment of intrusion and avoidance as well as measures of anxiety and depression. These two dimensions derive from work on traumatic events and assess the degree to which a woman is experiencing involuntary intrusions into her life such as thoughts or nightmares about the experience, together with how much she is actively avoiding people or situations which may re-evoke the experience. These two aspects are considered to be important indicators of the development and completion of the adaptational process through which an experience becomes fully incorporated into a person's sense of self. This work suggested that arriving at one's own explanation for why the miscarriage occurred, together with this leading to a general reappraisal of values in life (for example changing ones values to emphasize health and placing less emphasis on material goods), was associated with lower levels of intrusive thoughts. A belief in some sort of clear physical cause was associated with lower anxiety and a strong belief in personal control over the outcome of future pregnancies with higher anxiety levels. The fact that this study was completed upon a small sample must limit any conclusions which can be drawn but the potential relevance of such variables is demonstrated. It also seems that the information provided by staff about causation may, through influencing beliefs about causes, affect emotional adaptation. In particular the provision of information about medical causes may facilitate adjustment.

Implications and future directions

While a considerable number of studies have been conducted into different aspects of miscarriage, it is clear that there are still a number of gaps to be filled. The experiences of men whose partners have a miscarriage has not been systematically investigated, although it has been touched upon in, for example, Leroy (1988). In addition the effect on children and other family members has been given insufficient attention.

Our current knowledge concerning both the nature of the emotional consequences of miscarriage and factors which may predict more negative responses is clearly inadequate. In terms of considering predictors one weakness throughout this body of work is the failure of authors to use multivariate methods of analysis. The development of any predictive model requires progress beyond the separate consideration of each variable. In addition, the impact of aspects of the miscarriage experience, hospital and follow-up care processes and social support remain relatively unexplored and warrant detailed evaluation. In such studies it is important that the assessment of the care provided occurs as close as possible to the time of the experience and that the relationship with subsequent emotional response is assessed.

The nature of the hospital experience and support received from others may influence an individual's cognitive appraisal of the event. Cognitions about the miscarriage are likely to be influential mechanisms in determining emotional responses and yet have been given very little systematic consideration within the literature. There is now a considerable body of psychological investigation addressing the issue of coping with negative events (Taylor, 1983; Kiecolt-Glaser and Williams, 1987; Joseph, Brewin, Yule and Williams, 1991; Affleck and Tennen, 1991). This work has identified factors such as developing a personal understanding of the meaning and causation of an event as being important. In addition perceived control over recurrence, and thoughts designed to minimize the impact upon self esteem, may also influence emotional responses. These theories can constructively inform research in the field of coping with miscarriage and their incorporation should aid the development of useful predictive models.

All the studies referred to hitherto have been conducted within a broadly similar sociocultural environment, that is, they were all conducted within western developed societies. Socio-economic factors such as occupation and class were noted in some of the studies, as were age and parity. None of these studies, however, had attempted to explore what miscarriage means to women from diverse cultural backgrounds. One study which did so was that reported by Chalmers and Meyer (1992a, 1992b) which examined the psychosocial management and the emotional experience of miscarriage among four culturally different groups of women in South Africa. They found considerable cross-cultural variations in the emotions experienced by women, variations in coping patterns and differentiation in the availability and perceived value of people giving support. Reinharz (1988) attempted to locate the issue of miscarriage in a cross-cultural perspective by reviewing the literature that reports on miscarriage from a range of sociocultural (including historical) settings. Miscarriages clearly take place within an extremely diverse set of social and cultural, as well as technological and medical, contexts. The impact of a loss of a pregnancy is liable to vary according to differing culturally determined factors such as the gestational age at which a pregnancy is recognized (by the mother and by the society in question) and the stage at which the fetus/baby is attributed with human status.

Conclusion

In this chapter we have attempted to address a number of different aspects of miscarriage and have reported on some of the range of studies which have been undertaken in recent years. While the focus of the chapter has been 'miscarriage', at times we have been compelled, by the nature of the studies we have discussed, to refer also to stillbirth and early neonatal death. While other reproductive losses are discussed elsewhere in this volume it is inevitable that in this work, as in women's lives, there is no rigid demarcation between one type of reproductive loss and another. Pregnancy, as a continuum from the splitting of a cell to the birth of a new human being, can be disrupted or halted at virtually any stage, either voluntarily or involuntarily. Our focus here has been upon the stage of involuntary pregnancy loss known as miscarriage. Increased attention has been paid in recent years to the psychological and social factors associated with miscarriage. Nevertheless many aspects of both the immediate experience and the aftermath of a miscarriage, for the woman and her family still need to be understood. To this end we have attempted to indicate some of the areas upon which future research might fruitfully focus.

Applications

1. Individual reactions to miscarriage are very variable and are not simply related to the duration of the pregnancy. Sensitive care therefore requires to be tailored to the individual needs of the woman and her partner.

2. Providing information about the cause of miscarriage and its consequences for future pregnancies may ease distress and prevent harmful attributions and anxieties.

3. There is a need for follow-up, so information and support can be provided at appropriate times.

Further reading

Slade, P. (1994). Predicting the psychological impact of miscarriage. *Journal of Reproductive and Infant Psychology*, **12**, 5–16.
Moulder, C. (1990). *Miscarriage; Women's experiences and needs*. London: Pandora.

References

Abramson, L. Y., Metalsky, G. I. and Alloy, L. B. (1989). Hopelessness depression: a theory based subtype of depression. *Psychological Review*, **96**, 358–72.
Affleck, G. and Tennen, H. (1991). Appraisal and coping predictors of mother and child outcomes after newborn intensive care. *Journal of Social and Clinical Psychology*, **10**, 424–47.
Cecil, R. and Leslie, J. C. (1993). Early miscarriage: preliminary results from a study in Northern Ireland. *Journal of Reproductive and Infant Psychology*, **11**, 89–95.
Chalmers, B. (1992). Terminology used in early pregnancy loss. *British Journal of Obstetrics and Gynaecology*, **99**, 357–8.
Chalmers, B. and Meyer, D. (1992a). A cross-cultural view of the psychosocial management of miscarriage. *Journal of Psychosomatic Obstetrics and Gynaecology*, **13**, 163–76.
Chalmers, B. and Meyer, D. (1992b). A cross-cultural view of the emotional experience of miscarriage. *Journal of Psychosomatic Obstetrics and Gynaecology*, **13**, 177–86.
Charles, D. and Larsen, B. (1987). Infectious agents as a cause of spontaneous abortion. In *Spontaneous and Recurrent Abortion* (M. J. Bennett and D. K. Edmonds, eds). Oxford: Blackwell Scientific Publications.
Connolly, K. D. (1989). Factors affecting grief following pregnancy loss. In *The Free Woman: Women's Health in the 1990s* (E. V. Van Hall and W. Everaerd, eds). Carnforth: Parthenon.
Conway, K. (1992). Couples and fetal loss. *Journal of Psychosomatic Obstetrics and Gynaecology*, **13**, 187–95.
Cordle, C. J. and Prettyman, R. J. (1994). A 2-year follow-up of women who have experienced early miscarriage. *Journal of Reproductive and Infant Psychology*, **12**, 37–43.
Friedman, T. (1989). Women's experiences of general practitioner management of miscarriage. *Journal of the Royal College of General Practitioners*, **39**, 456–8.

Friedman, T. and Gath, D. (1989). The psychiatric consequences of spontaneous abortion. *British Journal of Psychiatry*, **155**, 810–13.

Garel, M., Blondel, B., Lelong, N., Papin, C., Bonenfaut, S. and Kaminiski, M. (1992). Réactions dépressives après une fausse couche. *Contraception, Fertility and Sexuality*, **20**, 75–81.

Graves, W. L. (1987). Psychological aspects of spontaneous abortion. In *Spontaneous and Recurrent Abortion* (M. J. Bennett and D. K. Edmonds, eds). Oxford: Blackwell Scientific Publications.

Hamilton, S. (1989). Should follow-up be provided after miscarriage? *British Journal of Obstetrics and Gynaecology*, **96**, 743–5.

Helstrom, L. and Victor, A. (1987). Information and emotional support for women after miscarriage. *Journal of Psychosomatic Obstetrics and Gynaecology*, **7**, 93–8.

Hey, V. (1989). A feminist exploration. In *Hidden Loss. Miscarriage and Ectopic Pregnancy* (V. Hey, C. Itzin, L. Saunders and M. Speakman, eds). London: The Woman's Press.

Hey, V., Itzin, C., Saunders, L. and Speakman, M. (eds) (1989). *Hidden Loss. Miscarriage and Ectopic Pregnancy*. London: The Woman's Press.

Horowitz, M. J. (1975). Intrusive and repetitive thoughts after experimental stress. *Archives of General Psychiatry*, **32**, 1457–83.

Jackman, C., McGee, H. M. and Turner, M. (1991). The experience and psychological impact of early miscarriage. *Irish Journal of Psychology*, **12**, 108–120.

Joseph, S. A., Brewin, C. R., Yule, W. and Williams, R. (1991). Causal attributions and psychiatric symptoms in survivors of the Herald of Free Enterprise Disaster. *British Journal of Psychiatry*, **159**, 542–6.

Kaplan, S. H., Greenfield, S. and Ware, J. E. jr (1989). Impact of the doctor–patient relationship on the outcomes of chronic disease. In *Communicating with Medical Patients* (M. Stewart and D. Roter, eds). Beverley Hills, CA: Sage.

Kiecolt-Glaser, J. K. and Williams, D. A. (1987). Self blame, compliance and distress among burn patients. *Journal of Personality and Social Psychology*, **53**, 187–93.

Kline, J. and Stein, Z. (1987). Epidemiology of chromosomal anomalies in spontaneous abortion: prevalence, manifestation and determinants. In *Spontaneous and Recurrent Abortion* (M. J. Bennett and D. K. Edmonds, eds). Oxford: Blackwell Scientific Publications.

Kohner, N. (1992). *A Dignified Ending*. London: SANDS.

Layne, L. L. (1990). Motherhood lost: Cultural dimensions of miscarriage and stillbirth in America. *Women and Health*, **16**, 69–98.

Layne, L. L. (1992). Of fetuses and angels: fragmentation and integration in narratives of pregnancy loss. In *Knowledge and society: The Anthropology of Science and Technology* (D. Hess and L. L. Layne, eds). Greenwich, CT: JAI Press Inc.

Lazarus, R. S. and Folkman, S. (1984). *Stress Appraisal and Coping*. New York: Springer.

Leppert, P. C. and Pahlka, B. S. (1984). Grieving characteristics after spontaneous abortion: a management approach. *Obstetrics and Gynaecology*, **64**, 119–22.

Leroy, M. (1988). *Miscarriage*. London: Macmillan Optima.

Lovell, A. (1983). Some questions of identity: late miscarriage, stillbirth and perinatal loss. *Social Science and Medicine*, **17**, 755–61.

Madden, M. E. (1988). Internal and external attributions following miscarriage. *Journal of Social and Clinical Psychology*, **7**, 113–21.

Moohan, J., Ashe, R. and Cecil, R. (1994). The management of miscarriage: results from a survey at one hospital. *Journal of Reproductive and Infant Psychology*, **12**, 17–19.

Moulder, C. (1990). *Miscarriage: Women's Experiences and Needs*. London: Pandora.

Neugebauer, R., Kline, J., O'Connor, P., Shrout, P., Johnson, J., Skodol, A., Wicks, J. and Susser, M. (1992). Depressive symptoms in women in the six months after miscarriage. *American Journal of Obstetrics and Gynaecology*, **166**, 104–109.

Oakley, A., McPherson, A. A. and Roberts, H. (1984). *Miscarriage*. Glasgow: Fontana.

Prettyman, R. J., Cordle, C. J. and Cook, G. D. (1993). A three month follow-up of psychological morbidity after early miscarriage. *British Journal of Medical Psychology*, **66**, 363–72.

Regan, L., Braude, P. R. and Trembath, P. L. (1989). Influence of past reproductive performance on risk of spontaneous abortion. *British Medical Journal*, **299**, 541.

Reinharz, S. (1988). Controlling women's lives: a cross-cultural interpretation of miscarriage accounts. In *Research in the Sociology of Health Care* (D. Wertz, ed.). Greenwich, CT: JAI Press Inc.

Roberts, H. (1989). A baby or the products of conception: lay and professional perspectives on miscarriage. In *The Free Woman: Women's Health in the 1990s* (E. V. Van Hall and W. Everaerd, eds). Carnforth: Parthenon.

Roberts, H. (1991). Managing miscarriage: the management of the emotional sequelae of miscarriage in training practices in the west of Scotland. *Family Practice*, **8**, 117–20.

Robinson, G. E., Stirtzinger, R., Stewart, D. E. and Ralevski, E. (1994). Psychological reactions in women followed for 1 year after miscarriage. *Journal of Reproductive and Infant Psychology*, **12**, 31–6.

Scherer, K. R. (1984). On the nature and function of emotion: a component processes approach. In *Approaches to Emotion* (K. R. Scherer and P. Ekman, eds). Hillsdale, NJ: Erlbaum.

Simpson, J. L. and Bombard, A. (1987). Chromosomal abnormalities in spontaneous abortion: frequency, pathology and genetic counselling. In *Spontaneous and Recurrent Abortion* (M. J. Bennett and D. K. Edmonds, eds). Oxford: Blackwell Scientific Publications.

Slade, P. (1994). Predicting the psychological impact of miscarriage. *Journal of Reproductive and Infant Psychology*, **12**, 5–16.

Slade, P. and Lee, C. (1995). Post traumatic stress and the consequences of miscarriage. Paper presented at British Psychological Society 1995 Conference, Warwick.

Slade, P. and Wills, G. (1993). Improving the quality of care for women experiencing early miscarriage. Report for Northern General Hospital Trust, Sheffield.

Stillbirth and Neonatal Death Society (SANDS) (1991). Guidelines for Professionals: Miscarriage, Stillbirth and Neonatal Death.

Statham, H. and Green, J. (1994). The effects of miscarriage and other 'unsuccessful' pregnancies on feelings early in a subsequent pregnancy. *Journal of Reproductive and Infant Psychology*, **12**, 45–54.

Stroebe, M. (1992–93). Coping with bereavement: a review of the grief work hypothesis. *OMEGA Journal of Death and Dying*, **26**, 19–42.

Taylor, S. E. (1983). Adjustment to negative events: a theory of cognitive adaptation. *American Psychologist*, **38**, 1161–73.

Teasdale, J. D. and Barnard, P. J. (1993). *Affect cognition and change.* Hillsdale, NJ: Erlbaum.

Tharpar, A. K. and Tharpar, A. (1992). Psychological sequelae of miscarriage: a controlled study using the general health questionnaire and the hospital anxiety and depression scale. *British Journal of General Practice*, **42**, 94–6.

Tunaley, J., Slade, P. and Duncan, S. B. (1993). Cognitive processes in psychological adaptation to miscarriage: a preliminary report. *Psychology and Health*, **8**, 369–81.

Van Gennep, A. (1909). *Les Rites de Passage.* Paris: Emile Nourry. *The Rites of Passage* (transl. M. B. Vizedom and G. L. Caffee) (1960). London: Routledge and Kegan Paul.

Warburton, D. and Strobino, B. (1987). Recurrent spontaneous abortion. In *Spontaneous and Recurrent Abortion* (M. J. Bennett and D. K. Edmonds, eds). London: Blackwell Scientific Publications.

Williams, J. M. G., Watts, F. N., Macleod, C. and Mathews, A. (1988). *Cognitive Psychology and Emotional Disorders.* Chichester: Wiley.

8

Antenatal preparation

Pauline Slade

In the UK considerable NHS resources are put into the provision of antenatal preparation for childbirth and parenthood. Large numbers of mothers and fathers-to-be spend substantial periods of time participating in these antenatal classes while smaller numbers choose to attend preparation sessions which they self-fund directly. In this chapter, Pauline Slade assesses the outcomes of antenatal preparation and points out the complexity of determining what constitutes a beneficial outcome, and on whom it confers benefit. Issues raised in this chapter are related to Chapter 9 on experiences of childbirth and Chapter 11 in its discussion of labour pain.

Introduction

Since the middle of this century antenatal preparation has been a feature of care during pregnancy. It was initially conceptualized as preparation for labour. Today in the United Kingdom the organization of classes varies considerably with some beginning in early pregnancy and focusing on matters such as self-care and hygiene and others taught later in pregnancy generally seeking to prepare women for labour and parenthood.

In Britain, antenatal classes are organized within the National Health Service, and, as documented by Combes and Schonveld (1992), provide women with information about pregnancy, the birth process and probable experiences that women will encounter. Specific techniques are often taught for coping with labour including breathing patterns, a variety of relaxation techniques and postural strategies. Typically a series of five to eight classes are organized on a weekly basis. In some places classes are run by midwives whilst in others responsibility is shared with obstetric physiotherapists who teach the coping strategies for labour. Often women are given a choice of attending 'women only' or 'couples' classes. Many specific initiatives have been introduced to encourage attendance from those still in their teens and from minority ethnic groups, as attendance at standard classes has been low. The actual classes themselves vary considerably in terms of their location, objectives, structure, the methods taught, and the qualifications of the instructors. Classes may take place in hospital ante-natal clinics or health centres in the community. A relatively recent innovation are aquanatal classes which are generally led by midwives at local leisure pools. Classes may promote or discourage decision-making, the use of medication in labour or acceptance of routine interventions.

As well as classes organized through the National Health Service, the Natural Childbirth Trust (NCT) is also an active provider of antenatal preparation. These classes are self-funding and therefore run on a fee-paying basis. Their content is not dissimilar to Health Service classes but there is often a particular emphasis on encouraging women and their partners to identify and work for the kind of birth they would like, developing techniques for pain reduction and sharing ideas and experiences in a group. The NCT has been viewed as a middle-class organization but there have recently been attempts to extend its work more to young women, single parents and ethnic minorities (NCT, 1991). The Active Birth Movement also runs antenatal classes in which the underlying philosophy is the importance of freedom of movement, instinctive behaviour and the selection of the best positions for labour (Williams and Booth, 1985). There are therefore a range of different preparation opportunities open to women during their pregnancies.

Not only do classes vary by organization, structure and content but women themselves attend for a variety of reasons. For many making contact with other women who will be having babies around the same time is important whilst others are more concerned with learning what to expect in labour and the post-partum (Hillier and Slade, 1989).

Theoretical bases for antenatal education

Read (1933) suggested that pain was experienced in labour because society has led women to expect this. He took the view that this expectation led to fear and that consequent tension in the uterine muscle fibres led to pain. He proposed that through education this cycle could be broken. If expectations could be changed through learning that muscular relaxation could relieve tension then the pain could also be relieved (see Chapter 11). In addition, breathing patterns taught antenatally could be used by women during labour to produce similar effects. A different theoretical basis underpins the process of psychoprophylaxis known as the Lamaze method, which incorporates a specified series of breathing levels. This is based on two principles to combat and eliminate pain: education of the mother and the conditioning of reflexes (Velvovsky, Platnov, Ploticher and Shugnom, 1960). It was suggested that the pain of labour could be bypassed by viewing uterine contractions as painful stimuli which could be inhibited or blocked by the development of new conditioned reflexes based upon breathing strategies. Both of these early theories suggest that the use of breathing or relaxation strategies will lead to a reduction in the experience of pain. Although today classes do not adhere specifically to either model, elements of these are still incorporated. There is no strong alternative conceptual framework in general use in Health Service settings.

Use of antenatal preparation strategies during labour

It is unclear whether women actually use the strategies they have been taught at classes when they are in labour. Copstick, Hayes, Taylor and Morris (1985) in a rare assessment of whether strategies were used concluded that it should no longer be assumed that women taught such techniques will necessarily be able to make use of them. This raises a question about how frequently training develops into actual practice. Slade, MacPherson, Hume and Maresh (1993) in their comparison of expectations and experiences reported that women expected to exert more control over their pain, to use their coping methods more and for them to be more effective than actually occurred. This suggests that many women may not translate preparation into practice. Similarly, Niven (1986) suggested that an association between antenatal class attendance and use of strategies existed only for relaxation methods.

Green (1993) reported results from a large study conducted by post. Questionnaires were given to women at 28–30 weeks' gestation, 4 weeks prior to the expected date of delivery and then finally at 6 weeks' postpartum. She found that most women intended to use breathing and relaxation exercises during labour (79%). Sixty-three per cent actually used breathing and relaxation exercises all or most of the time; 27% used them for a while and 10% did not use them at all. Overall in this study women found the exercises to be more useful than expected. Half found them very helpful and 5% found that the exercises allowed them to control the pain completely. Women who had said antenatally that they expected labour to be just moderately uncomfortable (i.e. a low point on the pain rating scale) were the most likely to use breathing and relaxation exercises and to find them very helpful. However, there was no assessment of attendance at antenatal preparation classes and therefore it was unclear how use related to this factor.

Another study which has considered what actually happens during labour is reported by Byrne-Lynch (1991). Women were asked about their use of coping strategies, medication and feelings of control. A high use of coping strategies was found with 95% in early labour, 76% in late first stage and 55% during transition. Walking and upright positions were the most commonly used strategy in early labour (65%). The next most popular was breathing exercises (33%). However only 20% of this sample had attended classes and therefore these findings relate mainly to spontaneously generated methods.

In summary, very little information is available about women's actual use of coping strategies during labour and how these are related to antenatal preparation.

Outcomes of antenatal education

There are approximately 700 000 births annually in England and Wales and in almost all of these women will have been offered some form of antenatal education. Attendance rates vary widely but Michie, Marteau and Kidd (1992) found that as many as 81% of women may attend at least one class. Considerable financial resources are allocated to this endeavour and an important question is whether participation leads to beneficial outcomes.

Assessing outcomes

The variations already noted in terms of content, duration and timing of classes, and expertise of staff create difficulties in comparability of outcome studies. In addition women who choose to attend classes may differ psychologically from those who choose not to attend and therefore comparisons may be based upon groups who differ in ways other than just their attendance at antenatal preparation classes. There is certainly evidence to suggest that demographically women who do attend may be significantly different from those who do not. For example, Bennett, Hewson, Booker and Holliday (1985) reported that frequent attenders were older and Michie, Marteau and Kidd (1992) found a positive social class bias. However, there may also be significant differences in coping attitudes, with non-attenders more likely to think that 'the less they knew about pregnancy and birth the better' (Michie, Marteau and Kidd, 1992). One final difficulty is that comparisons have generally been based upon whether women have attended or not attended classes and only on rare occasions has the number of hours of attendance been assessed.

Whether antenatal preparation leads to beneficial outcomes is a complex question since it involves defining *what* constitutes a beneficial outcome and for *whom*. One of the most basic aims is to provide information and there is some but not conclusive evidence that this is accomplished. Hillier and Slade (1989) assessed women's knowledge levels at the start of antenatal classes then assessed them again after the final class. Significant increases in knowledge were found after classes. However, women were self-selected in this study and there was no control group. Earlier studies utilized medication use as a measure of the effectiveness of classes on pain reduction, alongside other obstetric outcomes. More recent research has assessed psychological outcomes such as the emotional experience of labour and aspects of satisfaction. It therefore seems appropriate to consider in sequence a series of outcome variables and their relationship to antenatal preparation, relating firstly to the general area of pain in labour, and secondly to satisfaction with labour and psychological well-being.

Pain-related outcomes

One important pain-related outcome measure is the use of medication during labour. In order to provide some comparative data, only studies which have attempted to use some form of control group will be included here. One of the earliest reports was from Davis and Marrone (1962) who compared 355 self-selected prepared women with 108 women who had not attended classes. No differences were found between the two groups in terms of their use of analgesia or anaesthesia during labour and the authors comment upon the fact that motivation to take the classes may have a significant influence on results. Enkin, Smith, Dermer and Emmett (1972) addressed this issue by comparing women taking psychoprophylaxis classes with two control groups; women who wanted to attend but could not because the classes were full and a group of women drawn from the general population. Motivation to take classes had therefore been controlled between the trained group and the first control group. Trained women were found to use significantly less analgesia and anaesthesia than either of the control groups. No statistical differences were found between the two control groups, hence the reduced use of medication was attributed by the authors to the effects of training.

A study which tried to control for the effects of attendance in a different way was carried out by Timm (1979). Women were randomly assigned to one of three conditions: standard prenatal classes, knitting classes or no classes but encouragement to consult doctors or nurses about childbearing. Women who attended the prenatal classes used significantly less medication than those in the two control groups. It must be noted that the interpretation of randomized studies is often complicated by the fact that some participants will drop out, particularly, as in this case, if their allocated involvement has poor face validity.

Finally Hetherington (1990) in a controlled study compared 52 couples who attended childbirth classes with a control group matched for race, patient status, marital status, parity and age. Prepared couples were found to have more spontaneous deliveries as opposed to deliveries requiring specific assistance such as with forceps or by caesarean section. They also used less analgesia and anaesthesia. There were suggestions that the classes themselves may have helped women to cope with labour using less medication. In addition many of the couples attributed their satisfying birth experiences to the classes and felt that using methods taught during preparation had helped to achieve this. Better designed studies would seem therefore to suggest that women who have attended antenatal preparation do not use as much pain medication during labour.

It would be inappropriate to assume that reduced use of medication implies that women actually experience less severe pain. There are many factors which may influence women's use of pain relief in labour including hospital policy, availability of analgesia, quality of labour support and motivation of the mothers themselves to use or avoid drugs. There is a great deal of work to suggest that the experience of pain is related to multiple factors including sensory information, affective reactions and cognitive activity. The second and third factors may be influenced by individual psychological differences and aspects of the environment. The meaning attached to pain and the context in which it occurs can influence how it is experienced (Nettelbladt, Fagerstroim and Uddenberg, 1976).

Studies that have evaluated the pain women feel in labour suggest two main findings. Firstly, that the range of pain intensities that women experience is great. Secondly, that the average level of pain in labour is very high when considered on the spectrum of pain experiences in life (see Chapter 11). The influence of antenatal preparation on pain experience is addressed by many studies with conflicting results. A study by Davenport-Slack and Boylan (1974) illustrates the importance of the assessment measures used. They found that when women were asked to describe childbirth pain in relation to other painful experiences, 97% of women said childbirth was the most painful experience they had ever had. However when women rated their pain on a scale from 'extremely painful' to 'not painful at all' only 27% of women rated childbirth as extremely painful.

Melzack, Taenzer, Feldman and Kinch (1981) evaluated women's experience of pain in labour using the McGill Pain Questionnaire, for both women who had attended childbirth preparation classes and non-attenders. The average intensity of labour pain was very high with scores ranging from 'mild' to 'excruciating'. Labour was rated as more painful by primiparous women. However for primiparous women, childbirth training and practice were associated with lower ratings of pain. Studies by Charles, Morr, Block et al. (1978) and Brewin and Bradley (1982) similarly reported that attenders at classes rated their experience of labour as less painful. Beck, Siegel, Davidson et al. (1980) found participation in preparatory classes to be the best predictor of patient pain ratings, accounting for 20% of the variance.

However, other studies comparing the experiences of pain have failed to find any differences between class attenders and non-attenders (Slade, MacPherson, Hume and Maresh, 1993; Davenport-Slack and Boylan, 1974; Reading and Cox, 1985). While Niven and Gijsbers (1984) found no association between attendance at classes and total pain intensity ratings, there was some reduction in the affective dimension of pain and lower pain scores were reported by women who had previous experiences of significant levels of pain unrelated to child-birth. They concluded that these women may have already developed coping strategies that they then used to cope with pain during labour.

Bennet, Hewson, Booker and Holliday (1985) also failed to find any association between preparation and pain. Although this study is retrospective (a questionnaire was given to women at 3 weeks postpartum), it is of interest because, unlike others, attendance at childbirth preparation classes was measured not in terms of whether or not women attended but as the number of hours of classes they attended. Women who had attended more hours of classes used less medication and were more likely to use breathing techniques, verbal support and massage for pain relief, even though their reports of pain did not differ from women who had experienced fewer hours of preparation. In addition women who had attended more hours of classes were more likely to report that they had already planned not to take any medication for pain relief than medium, low, or non-attenders. If attendance at antenatal preparation itself does not reliably influence pain experiences are there other factors which may be related to antenatal preparation which do exert some influence?

Studies already cited indicate that previous experience of pain and the use of coping strategies may be important. Another study which suggests that attendance at classes may be a necessary but not sufficient condition to influence pain is reported by Wuitchik, Hesson and Bakal (1990). Pain was assessed during three stages of labour; latent (early), active and transition (approaching delivery) using the Present Pain Intensity Scale which involved a verbal rating of adjectives from 'no pain' to 'excruciating' and a visual analogue scale. Degree of practice and confidence in prepared childbirth techniques was assessed using a questionnaire given to women on arrival at the hospital. Confidence in their ability to use relaxation exercises was associated with reduced pain in latent but not active labour. Practice of breathing exercises was found to be related not to pain but to reduced distress in latent labour. Wuitchik, Hesson and Bakal (1990) reported that pain in latent labour was related to women's fear of pain, feelings of helplessness and loss of control. However this fear was also shown to be moderated by the practice of breathing exercises. Similar findings are reported by Lowe (1987).

In another report Wuitchik, Bakal and Lipshitz (1990) studied two groups of women: those who received an epidural (an injection of anaesthetic into the spine which removes feeling from the lower half of the body) during active labour and those who continued through three stages of labour: latent, active and transition, without an epidural. In the no analgesia group, subjective pain and distress-related cognition scores correlated significantly within the latent phase, but an association between pain and thought was not apparent during either the active or transition phase. Women who had received an epidural and were therefore devoid of pain continued to display distress-related thoughts.

The variability in findings about the influence of antenatal preparation on pain experience may occur because attendance acts as a facilitator of processes which may influence the experience of pain, such as confidence in coping, the actual use of strategies or low levels of fear of pain or distress-related cognitions. However, experience in labour can be enhanced through improved coping whilst the intensity of pain remains the same, not necessarily through a direct reduction in pain intensity. In addition, it is important to note that attenders and non-attenders at classes may have different expectations about their use of medication in labour with attenders possibly being more motivated to avoid analgesia. Any such lack of comparability between groups prior to attendance at preparation classes inevitably complicates the interpretation of findings.

Psychological outcomes

Antenatal preparation may influence other outcomes which are equally as important as the experience of pain, such as the emotional aspects of the experience of labour and satisfaction with this experience. Obstetrics has been mainly concerned with the amount of pain women experience in labour and has regarded this as central to a woman's overall experience. Thus, initially the major concern of antenatal education was with non-pharmaceutical reduction of pain in labour. However studies that have looked at women's satisfaction with the labour experience find little direct association between levels of pain and satisfaction (Morgan, Bulpitt, Clifton and Lewis, 1982). For example, Brewin and Bradley (1982) found that women who attended childbirth classes had less painful labours but their experiences were no more satisfying. Hence satisfaction with the childbirth experience may be independent of the pain felt. This is further confirmed by Salmon, Miller and Drew (1990) who interviewed women who had delivered healthy babies to identify the dimensions on which women evaluate their birth experiences. Two dimensions emerged: achievement concerned with such feelings as fulfilment; and pleasantness, a dimension of positive emotions. Ratings of painfulness did not show any loading on either component. However one difficulty with these measures is that the dimensions were conceptualized as bipolar, that is either as pleasant or unpleasant, fulfilling or unfulfilling whereas Slade, MacPherson, Hume and Maresh (1993) found that individuals' positive and negative dimensions were not inversely correlated and that it was important to consider dimensions independently.

It is clear that satisfaction with childbirth is not *directly* related to pain experience and there may be other important outcome dimensions against which antenatal preparation should be considered. This does not imply that the experience of pain is unimportant or preclude a more indirect relationship between pain and satisfaction which may be influenced by antenatal preparation. However it is clearly important that consideration is given to outcome variables other than pain.

Slade, MacPherson, Hume and Maresh (1993) specifically considered the impact of attendance at antenatal classes on the emotional experiences of labour. Eighty-one women giving birth to their first baby at a city centre teaching hospital were assessed. Ratings of expectations were made between 1 and 3 weeks before the expected date of delivery and experiences were assessed within 72 hours of labour. Sixty-two per cent of the sample had attended ante-natal classes. Three aspects of labour were addressed: emotional, medical and control variables, and women were asked about their attendance at childbirth preparation classes. Neither positive nor negative emotions experienced in labour differed between the groups. From this study attendance at, or number of childbirth preparation classes attended, showed little relationship with women's experience of labour contradicting an earlier study by Charles, Norr, Block et al. (1978) which suggested that attenders showed higher scores on an enjoyment index.

An important question is whether antenatal preparation influences satisfaction with labour. However, the concept of satisfaction is complex and many different aspects have been considered. One aspect of satisfaction is satisfaction with care. Green (1993) reported that satisfaction with care scores were related to the use of breathing and relaxation exercises and how helpful women found them to be. The most satisfied were women who used the exercises all of the time, followed by women who did not use them at all. The least satisfied were women who only used them for part of the time, hence those who said they only helped a bit or not at all were least satisfied. The more helpful women expected the exercises to be the more satisfied they were with labour.

Considering pain in relation to satisfaction, women who expected labour to be 'very' or 'unbearably' painful had lower satisfaction scores than those who did not expect the pain to be so bad. In addition these women were less satisfied both with how they coped with the pain and with the birth as a whole and also described themselves as significantly more out of control, frightened, powerless and helpless. They felt less in control of their contractions and of what staff were doing to them and in less control of their own behaviour. Those women who found labour pain to be exactly as expected were more satisfied than those who did not. High antenatal worry about labour pain was clearly unhelpful in promoting satisfaction.

Slade, MacPherson, Hume and Maresh (1993) considered personal satisfaction defined as satisfaction with self. This dimension was considered as it is important that the experience of labour should not undermine self-esteem and thereby the capacity to cope with the initial demands of the parenting role. Ability to control panic was found to be a very strong predictor of personal satisfaction. Use of exercises, in turn, strongly predicted ability to control panic. However attendance at antenatal preparation or number of classes or pain experienced held no direct predictive capacity for personal satisfaction. This finding suggests that satisfaction in childbirth was mainly related to feelings of control and coping with panic rather than the intensity of pain. However Slade, MacPherson, Hume and Maresh (1993) did find an indirect relationship between pain and satisfaction. Low levels of negative emotions were found to relate to ability to control feelings of panic. Negative emotions during labour were predicted by the worst pain level women experienced. Hence there may be some relationship between pain and satisfaction mediated by levels of negative emotions, use of coping strategies and ability to control panic. In addition efficacy of the exercises, personal control over pain and control over the use and efficacy of medication positively correlated with personal satisfaction.

Slade, MacPherson, Hume and Maresh (1993) suggest that antenatal preparation may translate into use of strategies for some women and hence to an enhanced sense of control. Byrne-Lynch (1991) compared women who felt in control during late first stage and transition and those who did not and found that only 19% of the 'in control' group reported using no definite strategy compared to 65% of the 'not in control' group. Women who felt 'in control' made significantly greater use of breathing in early labour. Ninety-five per cent of the sample stated that they felt in control during early labour. In addition the 'in control' group were likely to be using at least one type of coping strategy from the beginning of labour. For second stage labour the 'in control' group from the first stage were significantly more likely to feel in control during second stage than the 'not in control' group. This finding suggests that if a woman loses her sense of personal control then it may be difficult to regain as labour progresses. Use of coping strategies does appear to facilitate feelings of control.

It is clear that antenatal preparation may facilitate the use of coping strategies which have the potential to generate beneficial outcomes. Creating a sense of control, reducing fears of pain or distress-related thoughts would also appear to be helpful. However, it is important to note that attendance at classes does not automatically lead to clear benefits. It is of interest to consider why such benefits may not occur. Contemporary psychological theories may offer some insights into this issue.

Contributions from contemporary psychological theory

Antenatal preparation has received little attention from psychologists and has developed relatively independently from initiatives in health psychology. Recent developments in this emerging field make it unsurprising that perceived control should be indicated as an important factor in positive experiences of labour. As Slade, MacPherson, Hume and Maresh (1993) point out, psychological models of preparation for stressful events focus upon being able to predict events and on engendering a sense of control, with helplessness being associated with negative psychological outcomes. In addition, literature on psychological pain management suggests that pain-related thoughts can alter the experience of pain and vice versa (Philips, 1988). Distress-related thoughts have been identified as factors increasing pain but have been shown to be responsive to psychological intervention through the development and rehearsal of cognitive restructuring strategies. Factors identified as important in the experience of labour show considerable congruence with other stressful circumstances and factors which predict positive outcomes are already recognized within various psychological models.

Self-efficacy theory

Wardle (1983) reports just one of many studies indicating that giving people control may reduce experienced pain. However, there is some debate about whether exerting control or *believing* that one can exert control is actually more important. Litt (1988) suggests that the latter may be more important in labour and therefore self-efficacy theory (Bandura, 1977) may be of relevance. This suggests that a behaviour is more likely to occur in the presence of three expectancies: that the woman believes she has the ability to carry out the behaviour, that she thinks this will bring about certain outcomes and that she herself positively values these outcomes. In the context of methods for coping with labour, she must feel she has the ability to carry them out, that they will lead to certain outcomes such as reduced pain or more calmness, and she must value these outcomes for herself.

Confidence in one's own ability to implement coping strategies coupled with low levels of fear of pain may be important predictors of positive emotional and satisfaction outcomes and clearly may be facilitated by antenatal preparation. Confidence may also have an important role in the perception of pain during labour as more than half of the variance in early labour pain and one-third of active labour pain can be explained by the woman's confidence in her ability to cope (Lowe, 1987, 1989). In addition Crowe and von Baeyer (1989) found confidence in the ability to control pain reported by women after completing antenatal classes significantly predicted post-delivery reports of labour pain, although it must be noted that this was based upon a very small sample. Hence women who say they are more confident in their ability to cope with labour do seem to report less pain during labour. Walker and Erdman (1984) suggest women's confidence is significantly increased by childbirth education. Hillier and Slade (1989) also found that confidence in coping with labour increased after antenatal classes.

Lowe (1991) suggests that women develop self-efficacy expectancies about labour through different methods and sources. Past experiences are likely to play a role. A woman's self-efficacy may also be enhanced through experiences of coping with other painful stimuli. Niven and Gijsbers (1984) note that women who have experienced severe pain prior to childbirth show a decrease in the amount of pain felt during labour. They suggest that these women may have developed coping skills which they then transferred to the labour situation. Social learning theory suggest that self-efficacy can be enhanced by watching others' successful performances. Another source of information to women about their self-efficacy comes from physiological responses of autonomic arousal that occur when anticipating or experiencing a stressful event. Often such signs signal a feeling of failure. Symptoms common in labour such as rapid heart rate, nausea, flushing, fatigue and pain may undermine a woman's confidence through her assumption that she is not coping well. How women are taught to label these natural responses may have important implications for their feelings of confidence which in turn may influence their pain experiences as noted earlier.

In a limited application of the self-efficacy model, Manning and Wright (1983) assessed expectancies of the ability to control labour pain without medication, an outcome expectancy that non-medical pain control techniques lead to the ability to control the pain of labour and delivery without medication, and the importance of a medication-free labour and delivery. Data were collected at the end of classes, during early labour and in the first week postpartum. It was found that self-efficacy expectancies contributed more to the prediction of persistence in pain control techniques than did outcome expectancy or personal importance of a medication-free labour. Skill training in pain control, length of labour, type of delivery, past medication use for pain and locus of control were all unrelated to use of pain medication during labour or the percentage of time without pain medication. However, the amount of practice of pain control skills carried out was positively related to self-efficacy expectancies but not to use of medication during labour.

The study suggests that self-efficacy expectancies may mediate behaviour change. However medication use is a very narrow criterion to use as a measure of the behaviours needed to cope with the stress of childbirth. A wider consideration of all of the behaviours that are concerned with self-efficacy beliefs about coping with labour is required.

Conclusions

In general, the strategies taught at antenatal classes do seem helpful but we need to know much more about whether women actually use coping strategies during labour and what mediates their use. In addition it seems likely that beneficial effects are mediated through helping women to control feelings of panic. Antenatal preparation should attempt to target more specifically the development of feelings of confidence in the ability to use strategies. This may mean enhancing levels of practice, prompting and encouragement. A clear realistic picture of labour needs to be given with some attention being paid to the nature of the sensations that can be expected so that these will not be mislabelled and reduce confidence. The idea that a sense of control is important is certainly not new, however there has been little progress made in understanding the mechanisms through which such perceptions can be achieved. In addition it may be that other coping strategies can be developed, for example specifically emphasizing cognitive distraction to counteract distressing thoughts, or focusing and sensory transformation methods. Whether such cognitive strategies and the more traditional coping methods are of benefit only in early stages of labour is open to question given the findings of Wuitchik, Hesson and Bakal (1990) and Wuitchik, Bakal and Lipshitz (1990) and this clearly requires further evaluation. Currently, mere attendance at antenatal classes does not confer routine benefits other than reduced use of medication. Therefore ways of enhancing and generating more reliable positive impact need to be examined.

Applications

1. Role of midwives
If midwives are to play a more active role in prompting and giving positive feedback for the use of coping strategies, then awareness of when women are attempting to use these methods is very important. Bradley, Brewin and Duncan (1983) suggest that midwives may not always correctly identify these efforts and there needs to be more emphasis on clear communication between midwives and women in labour on these issues. In addition little is known about midwives' views about the value of coping methods; negative attitudes may adversely affect women's efforts. This is clearly an area that requires further investigation. There is also little information about the impact on midwives when a woman is using these methods since paradoxically this could leave midwives feeling passive and deskilled.

2. Influence upon partners and the infant
The emphasis in this chapter has been upon the mothers' experiences. The other individuals concerned in the experience of labour are the partner, if present, and the baby. There is little information about the impact of labour on partners or the effects of their participation in antenatal preparation. However, there is evidence to suggest that the presence of partners during labour is helpful particularly if this

provides the mother with support in the use of coping strategies (Copstick, Hayes, Taylor and Morris, 1986).

Antenatal education may possibly benefit the baby because less analgesia is used, and there is clearly potential for positive outcomes through a mother's enhanced psychological well-being. However, given the difficulties of showing direct gains to the mother herself, purely through attendance, established benefits for the infant cannot yet be conclusively demonstrated.

Further reading

Simkin, P. and Enkin, M. (1990). Antenatal classes. In *Effective Care in Pregnancy and Childbirth* (M. Enkin, M. J. N. C. Keirse and I. Chalmers, eds). London: Oxford University Press.

References

Bandura, A. (1977). Self-efficacy: Toward a unifying theory of behavioural change. *Psychological Review*, **84**, 191–215.

Beck, N. C., Siegel, L. J., Davidson, N. P., Kormeier, S., Breitenstein, A. and Hall, D. G. (1980). The prediction of pregnancy outcome: maternal preparation, anxiety and attitudinal sets. *Journal of Psychosomatic Research*, **24**, 343–51.

Bennett, A., Hewson, D., Booker, E. and Holliday, S. (1985). Antenatal preparation and labour support in relation to birth outcomes. *Birth*, **12**, 9–16.

Bradley, C., Brewin, C. R. and Duncan, S. L. B. (1983). Perceptions of labour: discrepancies between midwives' and patients' ratings. *British Journal of Obstetrics and Gynaecology*, **90**, 1176–9.

Brewin, C. and Bradley, C. (1982). Personal control and the experience of childbirth. *British Journal of Clinical Psychology*, **21**, 263–9.

Byrne-Lynch, A. (1991). Coping strategies, personal control and childbirth. *Irish Journal of Psychology*, **12**, 145–52.

Charles, A. G., Norr, K. L., Block, C. R., Meyering, S. and Meyers, E. (1978). Obstetric and psychological effects of psychoprophylactic for childbirth. *American Journal of Obstetrics and Gynaecology*, **131**, 44–52.

Combes, G. and Schonveld, A. (1992). Life will never be the same again. London: Health Education Authority.

Copstick, S. M., Hayes, R. W., Taylor, K. E. and Morris, N. F. (1985). A test of common assumptions regarding the use of antenatal training during labour. *Journal of Psychosomatic Research*, **29**, 215–18.

Copstick, S. M., Taylor, K. E., Hayes, R. and Morris, N. (1986). Partner support and the use of coping techniques in labour. *Journal of Psychosomatic Research*, **30**, 497–503.

Crowe, K. and von Baeyer, C. (1989). Predictors of positive childbirth experience. *Birth*, **16**, 59–63.

Davenport-Slack, B. and Boylan, D. H. (1974). Psychological correlates of childbirth programme. *American Journal of Obstetrics and Gynaecology*, **84**, 1196–201.

Davis, C. D. and Marrone, F. A. (1962). An objective evaluation of a prepared childbirth programme. *American Journal of Obstetrics and Gynaecology*, **84**, 1196–1201.

Enkin, M. W., Smith, S. L., Dermer, S. W. and Emmett, J. O. (1972). An adequately controlled study of the effectiveness of PPM training. In *Psychosomatic Medicine in Obstetrics and Gynaecology* (N. Morris, ed.). Basel: Karger.

Green, J. M. (1993). Expectations and experiences of pain in labour: Findings from a large prospective study. *Birth*, **20**, 65–72.

Hetherington, S. E. (1990). A controlled study of the effect of prepared childbirth classes on obstetric outcomes. *Birth*, **17**, 86–91.

Hillier, C. A. and Slade, P. (1989). The impact of antenatal classes on knowledge, anxiety and confidence in primiparous women. *Journal of Reproductive and Infant Psychology*, **7**, 3–13.

Litt, M. D. (1988). Self-efficacy and perceived control: Cognitive mediators of pain tolerance. *Personality and Social Psychology*, **57**, 149–60.

Lowe, N. K. (1987). Individual variation in childbirth pain. *Journal of Psychosomatic Obstetrics and Gynaecology*, **7**, 183–92.

Lowe, N. K. (1989). Explaining the pain of active labour. The importance of maternal confidence. *Research in Nursing and Health*, **12**, 237–45.

Lowe, N. K. (1991). Maternal confidence in coping with labour. A self-efficacy concept. *Journal of Gynaecological and Neonatal Nursing*, **20**, 457–3.

Manning, M. M. and Wright, T. L. (1983). Self-efficacy expectancies, outcome expectancies, and the persistence of pain control in childbirth. *Journal of Personality and Social Psychology*, **45**, 421–31.

Melzack, R., Taenzer, P., Feldman, P. and Kinch, R. A. (1981). Labour is still painful after prepared childbirth training. *Canadian Medical Association Journal*, **125**, 357–63.

Michie, S., Marteau, T. M. and Kidd, J. (1992). Predicting antenatal class attendance: Attitudes of self and others. *Psychology and Health*, **7**, 225–34.

Morgan, B. M., Bulpitt, C. J., Clifton, P. and Lewis, P. J. (1982). Analgesia and satisfaction in childbirth (The Queen Charlottes' 1000 mother survey). *Lancet*, **2**, 808–11.

Natural Childbirth Trust (1991). NCT Teachers Annual Returns (1990) Outreach. London: Natural Childbirth Trust.

Nettelbladt, P., Fagerstroim, C. F. and Uddenberg, N. (1976). The significance of reported childbirth pain. *Journal of Psychosomatic Research*, **20**, 215–21.

Niven, C. (1986). Factors affecting labour pain. University of Stirling (unpublished doctoral thesis).

Niven, C. and Gijsbers, K. (1984). Obstetric and non-obstetric factors related to labour pain. *Journal of Reproductive and Infant Psychology*, **2**, 61–78.

Philips, H. C. (1988). The psychological management of chronic pain. New York: Springer.

Read, G. (1933). Natural childbirth. London: William Heinemann.

Reading, A. E. and Cox, D. N. (1985). Psychosocial predictors of labour pain. *Pain*, **2**, 309–15.

Salmon, P., Miller, R. and Drew, N. C. (1990). Women's anticipation and experience of childbirth: The independence of fulfilment, unpleasantness and pain. *British Journal of Medical Psychology*, **63**, 255–9.

Slade, P., MacPherson, S. A., Hume, A. and Maresh, M. (1993). Expectations, experiences and satisfaction with labour. *British Journal of Clinical Psychology*, **32**, 469–83.

Timm, M. M. (1979). Prenatal education evaluation. *Nursing Research*, **28**, 388–92.

Velvovsky, I., Platnov, K., Ploticher, V. and Shugnom, E. (1960). Painless childbirth through psychoprophylaxis. Moscow: Foreign Language Publishing House.

Walker, B. and Erdman, A. (1984). Childbirth Education Knowledge. *Birth*, **11**, 103–8.

Wardle, J. (1983). Psychological management of anxiety and pain during dental treatment. *Journal of Psychosomatic Research*, **27**, 399–402.

Williams, M. and Booth, D. (1985). Antenatal education guidelines for teachers. Edinburgh: Churchill Livingstone.

Wuitchik, M., Hesson, and Bakal, D. A. (1990). Perinatal predictors of pain and distress during labour. *Birth*, **17**, 186–91.

Wuitchik, M., Bakal, D. and Lipshitz, J. (1990). Relationships between pain, cognitive activity and epidural analgesia during labour. *Pain*, **41**, 125–32.

9

Birth experiences[1]

Lyn Quine and Derek Rutter
with an introduction by Catherine Niven

This short chapter introduces the topic of birth, being the first of three chapters dealing with different aspects of parturition. Birth experiences vary tremendously being graphically described by mothers in glowing or traumatic terms: 'It was like shelling peas'; 'it was like shitting a melon' or sometimes as both at the same time – 'it was the most wonderful experience of my entire life, it was like a red hot poker going through my spine'. Traditionally, the literature of childbirth has focused on either the physical survival and well being of the mother and child or on labour pain. In this chapter Lyn Quine and Derek Rutter report on the findings of a study on women's satisfaction with the quality of the birth experience, an approach which thereby focuses our attention on this central but frequently neglected aspect of birth.

Introduction

In our society childbirth is typically a medicalized event, usually taking place in hospital or at least attended by health care practitioners (see Chapter 4). In the UK, debate surrounding birth experiences is typically limited to the consideration of the extent of medical intervention and the most appropriate setting for birth; hospital, home or birth centre (e.g., Kitzinger, 1962; Tew, 1990). Our view of childbirth has been so clearly shaped by this that it is difficult for us to contemplate the true range of childbirth experiences that are possible. Variation in birth experience is, however, fundamental and extensive.

In biological terms there is only one certainty about the process of childbirth: once initiated, it can only end in the birth of a baby or the death of the mother. (In this context it is salutory to remember that over the centuries, countless women have died in childbirth. Safe childbirth is a very recent phenomenon and is restricted to a small proportion of the world's population.) Every other aspect of the process can vary – when labour occurs, how long it lasts, what sex the baby is, how many there are, how big they are, what the mother's dimensions are, how efficiently her labour progresses, etc. While technological developments have allowed some degree of predictability, for example in regard to the number and sex of babies, much remains unpredictable and the permutations of biological variability are endless.

Birth is more than a biological event however, and all birth experiences take place in a cultural context and are shaped by the views and practices of that

[1] This chapter is largely drawn from Quine, L., Rutter, D. R., Gowen, S. (1993). Women's satisfaction with the quality of the birth experience. *Journal of Reproductive Psychology*, **11** (2), 107–15. It is reproduced here with the kind permission of the *Journal of Reproductive Psychology*.

culture. Joan Raphael-Leff (1991) has recently provided a fascinating review of cultural variation in birth practices describing an incredible variety of birth experiences: from women who are segregated from society while giving birth, to those for whom birth is a publicly witnessed and celebrated event; from societies where the labouring woman is seen to have supernatural powers to those where she is regarded as dangerous, dirty or defiled. The mother may be assisted by other women, by male partners or by specialized attendants who have health care, social, and/or religious roles. These attendants can provide various sorts of practical, emotional or spiritual support; engage in sensory stimulation involving diverse stimuli including chanting, touch, incense or lewd banter; administer herbal remedies or poultices to ease discomfort or speed up labour; supply nourishment; and prescribe postures, aids and interventions which are designed to correct complications occurring during birth and facilitate delivery. Her review concludes that it is impossible to talk of a truly 'natural childbirth'. The human birth experience is always going to be influenced by practices and interventions which are a product of culture as well as nature.

In our own culture, many of the differences elucidated by anthropological research are also apparent. For example at various times childbirth has been a home-based semi-public event; a secret event taking place within the confines of hospital; an event from which fathers were banned and at which now their attendance is almost mandatory. Similarly, attitudes towards birth in our multi-cultural and diverse society are influenced by the cultural and religious back-ground of the mother, her family and obstetric staff in ways which are seldom acknowledged. Add to these sources of variability those derived from the professional considerations of the staff involved and the setting in which their involvement takes place; hi-tech, versus 'natural', consultant-run versus midwife-run, stainless steel trolleys versus bean bags and birthing pools, and the range of possible birth experiences within a single culture become endless.

As psychologists we are interested not just in variability in birth experiences per se but in the woman's reactions to and feelings about her particular birth experience. A number of books and papers have detailed women's reports of their birth experiences (see Further reading). This work provides us with a rich source of first-hand data about birth experiences to set alongside that derived from anthropological and biomedical research. A complementary approach is to examine the woman's own perceptions of her experience utilizing more structured assessments of psychological outcome. In the remainder of this chapter Lyn Quine and Derek Rutter take this approach in looking at some sociodemographic sources of variability and at the effects of the sociopsychological factors of social support and life events on women's satisfaction with the birth experience.

Women's satisfaction with the quality of the birth experience

The quality of a woman's childbirth experience is vital to her own well-being and to her future relationship with her partner and child (Doering, Entwisle and Quinlan, 1980). Childbirth has been viewed as a stressful life event (Chertok, 1966) but evidence suggests it can be mediated by social and psychological resources. For example Henneborn and Cogan (1975) and Norr, Block, Charles et al. (1977) have reported that both preparation for birth and partner participation have a positive effect upon the quality of childbirth, although the mechanisms that mediate between preparation and quality were not elucidated. Similarly it has been argued that the effect of stressful life events can be buffered by social support, either by reducing the effects of stress itself or by increasing an individual's coping strategies (Nuckolls, Cassel and Kaplan, 1972; Dimsdale, Eckenrode, Haggerty et al., 1979). Other demographic and psychosocial variables that may affect the quality of the woman's birth experience include age (Norr, Block, Charles et al., 1977), social class (Nelson, 1983; McIntosh, 1989), expectations and experience of pain (Norr, Block, Charles et al., 1977; Doering, Entwisle and Quinlan, 1980), and personal control (Green, Coupland and Kitzinger, 1990).

Rutter and Quine (1990) have produced a model of the role played in pregnancy outcome by sociodemographic factors such as age, marital status and social class, and social psychological variables such as social support and life events. This suggests that social psychological variables are best seen as mediators between sociodemographic factors, which they call social inputs, and pregnancy outcome. This model can be adapted to explain the significance of social inputs and social psychological mediators for women's satisfaction with the quality of their birth experience. In this case, social inputs include factors such as social class and age, while mediators might be social support, preparation for the birth, information about childbirth, locus of control and expectations and experience of pain.

Quine, Rutter and Gowen (1993) tested this model in a prospective study of 59 first-time mothers-to-be. The women were interviewed twice, towards the end of their pregnancies and again after the birth of their babies, to determine their satisfaction with the quality of the birth experience. Measures of preparation for childbirth, satisfaction with information, social support, expected pain and health locus of control were taken at the first interview and measures of social support, reported pain, symptoms of stress, reports of the baby's behaviour, and satisfaction with the birth were taken at the second interview.

In this study, working-class women were less satisfied with the experience of birth they had had than middle-class women. They also felt that they had been less well prepared for childbirth and were less satisfied with the information they had received about childbirth than middle-class women. Women who felt that they had been well informed about the childbirth also felt better prepared for it, and reported higher levels of satisfaction with the birth experience than those women who felt that they did not know what to expect. Middle-class women felt better supported by their partners, family and neighbours than did working-class women. Path analysis of the data showed that social class significantly affected both social support and information. However, regardless of social class, women who felt well supported at the end of their pregnancy reported less pain during the birth, and women who felt less pain reported greater satisfaction with the birth experience. This study also found that women who were satisfied with the birth experience reported fewer symptoms of stress when they were interviewed after the birth, and were more likely to describe their child's behaviour in positive terms. This study suggests that both social support and adequate information about childbirth act as mediators between social class and the experience of childbirth. Working-class women seem to be disadvantaged in both respects: they are less well supported than middle-class women, and they lack information about childbirth. As a result, they are less likely to find childbirth a rewarding experience.

Intervention studies in which women have been offered social support during both pregnancy and labour typically find that it has positive effects (Sosa, Kennell, Klaus et al., 1980; Oakley, Rajan and Grant, 1990). These effects include fewer admissions to hospital during pregnancy, shorter labours, greater awareness during delivery, less use of neonatal intensive care by babies, greater health service use by mothers and babies after the birth and improved psychological well-being, especially a reduction in anxiety. As Oakley and Rajan (1991) observe, the conventional picture of close-knit supportive social networks based on kin and neighbourhood among working-class women, reported in studies in the 1950s, is not borne out in later studies. Working-class women often lack social and emotional support and that is one reason why they may end up dissatisfied with the birth experience, since women who are supported feel less pain. Oakley and Rajan's analysis of obstetrically 'at risk' mothers showed that working-class women were 'less enmeshed in potentially helpful patterns of sociability than their middle-class counterparts' – they perceived themselves to have lower close contact with friends and relatives, were in contact with significant others less frequently, and derived less help and support from those relationships than did middle-class women. They also received less help, interest and emotional support from their male partners. Oakley and Rajan found that men living with working-class women were less likely to be said by their female partners to show an interest in the pregnancy, to take time off in pregnancy, to be with their partners, to accompany their partners to the clinic, to be present during labour and delivery, to change the baby's nappies, or to help with other children. As to what types of social support women most valued, Oakley and Rajan's research indicated that emotional support and company were thought to be most important, followed by help with child care.

A second reason for dissatisfaction is that women often feel that they have inadequate information and are unprepared for childbirth (Quine, Rutter and Gowen, 1993). There are many reasons why this may be the case. Firstly, there are problems of memory and comprehension. Many women, particularly working-class women, find the information given at antenatal classes difficult to remember and understand (see Chapter 8). Ley's influential research into doctor–patient communication argues that satisfaction and compliance with medical communications are dependent on both understanding and memory (Ley, 1988). If patients understand and remember what they are told they are more likely to be satisfied with the information and to comply with the doctor's advice. Ley suggests that patients' failures to understand stem from three inter-related problems. First, material may be presented to patients in a way which is difficult to understand. Second, materials may assume a knowledge of basic physiology or anatomy or an elementary medical knowledge about the human body which some patients do not have; and third, some patients may have misconceptions about their condition which interfere with their comprehension of the information given by the health professional. These factors may also be important in antenatal education.

Applications

The research in this area highlights a number of issues for policy and practice. First, women benefit from clear information which they are given during pregnancy. Health professionals may need training to improve their communications, perhaps giving consideration both to the content and style of what is said. Second, a number of studies have found that intervening to increase support during labour and delivery has positive effects (Sosa, Kennell, Klaus et al., 1980; Elbourne, Oakley and Chalmers, 1989; Oakley and Rajan, 1991). The results of Quine, Rutter and Gowan (1993) suggest that working-class women would particularly benefit from better social support. Thirdly, especially for first-time mothers, the quality of the childbirth experience may have far-reaching effects both on their stress levels during the first weeks after birth and their relationship with a new baby (Doering, Entwisle and Quinlan, 1980). If satisfaction can be increased, longer-term complications may well diminish.

Further reading

Kitzinger, S. (1966). *The Experience of Childbirth*. London: Golancz.

Raphael-Leff, J. (1991). *Psychological Processes of Childbearing*. London: Chapman and Hall.

Woollett, A. and Dosanjh-Matwala, N. (1990). Asian women's experiences of childbirth in East London: the support of fathers and female relatives. *Journal of Reproductive and Infant Psychology*, **8**, 11-23.

References

Chertok, L. (1966). *Motherhood and personality*. London: Tavistock.

Dimsdale, J. E., Eckenrode, J., Haggerty, R. J., Kaplan, B. H., Cohen, F. and Dornbusch, S. (1979). The role of social support in medical care. *Social Psychiatry*, **14**, 175–80.

Doering, S. G., Entwisle, D. R. and Quinlan, D. (1980). Modeling the quality of women's birth experience. *Journal of Health and Social Behaviour*, **21**, 12–21.

Elbourne, D., Oakley, A. and Chalmers, I. (1989). Social and psychological support during pregnancy. In *Effective Care During Pregnancy and Childbirth*, Volume 1: Pregnancy (I. Chalmers, M. Enkin and M. J. N. C. Keirse, eds). Oxford: Oxford University Press.

Green, J., Coupland, V. and Kitzinger, J. (1990). Expectations, experiences, and psychological outcomes of childbirth: a prospective study of 825 women. *Birth*, **17**, 15–24.

Henneborn, W. J. and Cogan, R. (1975). The effect of husband participation on reported pain and probability of medication during labour and birth. *Journal of Psychosomatic Research*, **19**, 215–22.

Kitzinger, S. (1962). *The Experience of Childbirth*. London: Golancz.

Ley, P. (1988). *Communicating with Patients*. London: Chapman and Hall.

Martin, J. and Roberts, C. (1984). *Women and Employment*. London: OPCS.

McIntosh, J. (1989). Models of childbirth and social class: a study of 80 working-class primagravidae. In *Midwives, Research and Childbirth* Volume 1. (S. Robertson and A. M. Thomson, eds). London: Chapman and Hall.

Nelson, M. (1983). Working-class women, middle-class women and models of childbirth. *Social Problems*, **30**, 284–97.

Norr, K. L., Block, C. R., Charles, A., Meyering, S. and Meyers, E. (1977). Explaining pain and enjoyment in childbirth. *Journal of Health and Social Behaviour*, **18**, 260–75.

Nuckolls, K. B., Cassel, J. and Kaplan, B. H. (1972). Psychosocial assets, life crisis and the prognosis of pregnancy. *American Journal of Epidemiology*, **95**, 431–41.

Oakley, A. and Rajan, L. (1991). Social class and social support: the same or different? *Sociology*, **25**, 31–59.

Oakley, A., Rajan, L. and Grant, A. (1990). Social support and pregnancy outcome. *British Journal of Obstetrics and Gynaecology*, **97**, 155–62.

Quine, L., Rutter, D. R. and Gowen, S. (1993). 'Women's satisfaction with the quality of the birth experience'. *Journal of Reproductive Psychology*, **11** (2), 107–15.

Raphael-Leff, J. (1991). *Psychological Processes of Childbearing*. London: Chapman and Hall.

Rutter, D. R. and Quine, L. (1990). Inequalities in pregnancy outcome: a review of psychosocial and behavioural mediators. *Social Science and Medicine*, **30**, 553–68.

Sosa, R., Kennell, J., Klaus, M., Robertson, S. and Urrutia, J. (1980). The effect of a supportive companion on perinatal problems, length of labour and mother–infant interaction. *New England Journal of Medicine*, **303**, 597–600.

Tew, M. (1990). *Safer Childbirth? A Critical History of Maternity Care*. London: Chapman and Hall.

Wallston, K. A. and Wallston, B. S. (1978). Development of the multidimensional health locus of control (MHLC) scale. *Health Education Monographs*, **6**, 160–70.

10

Caesarean section

Edith Hillan

One variety of birth experience is that of caesarean section, a procedure which is becoming increasingly common in this country. In this chapter, Edith Hillan debates the possible reasons for the increase, including clinical and non-clinical considerations, many of which are related to psychosocial factors as opposed to purely biological ones. The physical and psychosocial morbidity associated with caesarean section is discussed and is offset by data which shows the benefits of delivering a baby in this manner.

This chapter deals with antenatal preparation and is therefore linked to the material presented in Chapter 8. It also raises the topic of postnatal sexual adjustment which will be further considered in Volume 3 of the series.

Introduction

The incidence of both elective (performed *before* the onset of labour) and emergency (performed *after* the onset of labour) caesarean section has risen steadily in most developed countries over the last 20 years. Professional and lay concern about the spiral in caesarean section rates has prompted national reviews in an effort to establish the reasons for this upward trend (Rosen, 1981; Francome, Savage, Churchill and Lewison, 1993). The most dramatic increase in rates has occurred in the United States where one in four women now deliver their babies by caesarean section. Although the incidence of caesarean section is lower in the United Kingdom than the USA, the upward trend in the rate is still marked from 4.9% in 1970 to 14.0% in 1992 (Francome, Savage, Churchill and Lewison, 1993). The rate varies widely between hospitals – in a national survey of England and Wales in 1992 Francome and colleagues (1993) found the section rate ranged from 6.2% to 21.5% – and although there are demographic differences in the hospital populations they do not nearly account for such variations. This suggests that there must be marked differences in clinical practice.

The reasons for the increased use of caesarean section are complex. Until recent decades caesarean section was usually used as a last resort because of the high maternal mortality and morbidity associated with the operation. The introduction of antibiotics and blood transfusions as well as markedly improved anaesthetic and surgical techniques overcame the problem of shock, sepsis and haemorrhage often associated with caesarean delivery. As the maternal mortality rate reduced, doctors began to focus their attention on reducing perinatal loss and eventually the joint effort of obstetricians and paediatricians concentrated on reducing perinatal morbidity as well. This effort to improve the outcome of pregnancy is evidenced in part by the rise in the number and availability of neonatal intensive care units and the growth in the new interest area of perinatal medicine which has resulted in changes in clinical management and a huge increase in ante- and intrapartum fetal monitoring. The result of this has been rapidly improved survival rates and long-term outcomes for both mothers and infants at risk. At present in the United Kingdom a *pregnancy related* maternal death occurs once in every 17 500 deliveries and less than 8 babies in every 1 000 are either stillborn or die in the first week of life (Hall, 1995).

The clinical indications mainly responsible for the rise in caesarean section rates are now well described – dystocia (the term commonly used to encompass all those factors which cause labour to be prolonged, e.g. cephalopelvic disproportion, failure to progress in labour, failed induction, uterine hyper or hypotonia and cervical stenosis), repeat caesarean section, breech presentation and fetal distress (Rosen, 1981). However, there is a lack of available evidence to support the use of abdominal delivery for many of these common indications which led one obstetrician to comment that the increasing caesarean section rate 'is the result of one of the least controlled clinical experiments that has occurred in medicine' (Pearson, 1984).

Few studies have addressed the importance of non-clinical variables in decisions to deliver by caesarean section. In the USA, failure to perform a caesarean section is one of the commonest reasons for litigation and although malpractice suits are much less common in the UK, fear of litigation was the most common reason given by obstetricians in a British survey for the increased use of the operation (Francome, Savage, Churchill and Lewison, 1993). Other factors may include the loss of clinical skills in vaginal delivery of breech presentations, interpretation of the results of technology such as electronic fetal monitoring, economic factors, the available facilities and staffing within maternity units and individual consultant's policy. It is also notoriously difficult to reverse any established trend in medical practice because of the desire to conform to peer practice.

Attempts to justify the increase are usually made by linking caesarean section rates with perinatal mortality statistics. Although it is debatable whether there is a causal relationship between the current improvement in perinatal outcome and the increased use of caesarean section, the fact that many people both within and outwith the obstetric profession assume that there is, has probably influenced clinical decisions about the mode of delivery. It is interesting to note that whereas patterns of caesarean section rates differ both on national and international levels, the decrease in perinatal mortality rates is universal. Illustrative of this is the situation in a regional hospital in Dublin (O'Driscoll and Foley, 1983) and in a whole country, the Netherlands (Thiery and Derom, 1986) where, despite stable caesarean section rates, the perinatal outcome has improved to the same degree as in countries where caesarean rates have increased.

Morbidity associated with caesarean delivery

Although caesarean delivery is now safer than it has ever been, it remains a major surgical procedure and therefore can never be an entirely safe alternative to vaginal delivery. The NIH task force report (Rosen, 1981) estimated that the maternal mortality associated with caesarean section was four times greater than that associated with vaginal delivery and maternal morbidity rates were also greatly increased when delivery was effected by the abdominal route. However, definitions of morbidity lack uniformity and this in turn makes the classification of major and minor complications difficult, so any comparison of morbidity rates is of dubious value. Nevertheless there can be no doubt that morbidity is greater following caesarean delivery than after vaginal delivery. In a large-scale study which looked at the short-term morbidity associated with the operation it was found that three months after delivery, 35% of women still did not feel back to normal and 28% felt less healthy than before the pregnancy. The most common complaints following caesarean section were wound pain, wound leakage, tiredness, backache, constipation, depression and sleeping difficulties (Hillan, 1992a).

Most research related to the outcome of caesarean section has focused on assessment of the maternal and perinatal mortality and morbidity associated with the operation. However, childbirth is a social and personal experience as well as a medical event and for most women a satisfactory pregnancy outcome involves delivery of a healthy baby and a good childbirth experience.

Psychosocial outcomes

Few women today view pregnancy and delivery as a series of biological events over which they have no control, and, increasingly consumers are demanding a more humanistic approach to obstetric care and a greater share of responsibility in decision-making related to the care that they receive.

This increase in interest in the quality of childbirth can be seen in the amount of attention paid to pregnancy and delivery in the lay press and also in the realization by professionals of the importance of the delivery experience and early parent–infant bonding in establishing the family unit. The work of Klaus, Jerauld, Kreger et al. (1972) and Kennel, Jerauld, Wolfe et al. (1974) among others, though challenged by some, has indicated that early prolonged separation of the mother and her baby hampers the attachment process and may play a part in later parenting difficulties. The recent report of the Expert Maternity Group, Changing Childbirth (HMSO, 1993) stated that the woman must be the focus of maternity care. She should be able to feel that she is control of what is happening to her and able to make decisions about her care having discussed matters fully with professionals involved. The report also emphasized the importance of women being involved in the evaluation of the services provided to ensure thay they are responsive to the needs of women and of a changing society.

One problem in trying to measure satisfaction with maternity care is that no standardized or validated scales exist for doing so. Just as the recipients of perinatal care are not a homogeneous group, satisfaction will inevitably mean different things to different women. Satisfaction may also be dependent on a number of other factors including the maternal personality, the amount of preparation received before delivery, prior expectations of childbirth, past childbirth experience, the type of delivery and the degree of control a woman feels she has over her experience. A further difficulty in assessing satisfaction with care is that it is unstable and changes according to unrelated variables such as the woman's mood at the time of the interview, who is asking the questions, how the questions are posed and how much time has elapsed after the event (Shearer, 1983).

Pregnancy, childbirth and parenthood require massive physiological and psychological adjustments on the part of the woman. Even under normal circumstances the transition to motherhood may be problematical especially if the woman's prior expectations of her delivery do not meet up with the reality. Oakley (1980) found that the most normal of births can involve elements of loss for the mother – loss of self-confidence, loss of body image, loss of previous employment and so on. She states that:

> Childbirth is a life event with considerable loss and uncertain gain. The response is liable to be hopelessness and the extent of this is determined in large part by the extent to which people feel able to take control over their own lives.

In addition to these *normal* stressors, the woman who has had a caesarean section has to cope with the physical and psychological impact of anaesthesia and major surgery, which may have occurred on top of a long and exhausting labour.

Oakley (1983) commented on the difference in the way that caesarean section is conceptualized from other types of abdominal surgery. The term section is used as opposed to surgery or operation and this is associated with a difference in the way in which the effects of caesarean section and other surgical procedures are seen. A common generally accepted consequence of major surgery is depression, yet the same assumption is not made about caesarean section. Similarly, many of the general after-effects of surgery are applicable to caesarean section. These may include a temporary response of emotional relief and elation from having recovered from the anaesthetic, worry about the mutilating effects of the surgery and an extended period of physical and psychological discomfort (Janis, 1958). In addition, the woman who has experienced caesarean delivery is often expected to cope with the demands of her new baby and this may involve activities that are normally forbidden to patients that have undergone abdominal surgery.

During the same period that parents' expectations of childbirth have altered, there has been a steady rise in the caesarean section rate – especially in the numbers of woman having a first (primary) emergency section performed. This is important because if women are delivered by caesarean section they are much more likely to have this type of delivery in a subsequent pregnancy (repeat caesarean). Few women, unless alerted by obstetricians or by their previous obstetric history, seriously consider the possibility that they will require a caesarean section. As women have become increasingly actively involved in their pregnancies by reading more about childbirth and attending antenatal preparation classes, their expectations are chanelled towards a natural outcome of labour, where the mother is in control throughout and experiences a sense of fulfilment at the time of birth. The inevitable corollary to this is a parallel increase in disappointment if the birth events do not go as planned.

To date very little research has been carried out that has attempted to evaluate the psychosocial effects of caesarean delivery. This may be because until recently both parents and professionals accepted that caesarean section was only carried out as a life saving procedure. Few women doubt that the operation is only carried out in cases of *real* need when there is a risk for either the mother or her baby. If it is suggested to a woman that caesarean section is the best option for either herself or more significantly her baby, then not surprisingly she will be glad to have the operation. Certainly in Hillan's study (1992b) none of the women delivered by emergency caesarean section who were interviewed questioned the need for the operation, although many wanted more information about the events that had led up to it. One of the worrying findings of this study was that 13% of the women did not know or gave completely wrong explanations for the performance of the caesarean section and a further 14% were only partially right in their comprehension (Hillan, 1992a).

Emotional responses to caesarean delivery

Most of the studies which have examined parental responses to caesarean section have come from North America and are primarily descriptive in nature. By and large, they involve small study numbers and are confined to middle-class, Caucasian families who were self-selected from caesarean support groups. These self-help groups offer psychological and social support for women who have experienced caesarean delivery and their numbers have grown rapidly in the USA and to a lesser extent the United Kingdom. One interesting aspect of these groups is that they have voiced little criticism about the rising caesarean section rates, which implies that the recipients of such surgery tend to view it as being necessary.

One of the first studies to comment on mothers' views of caesarean delivery was reported by Affonso and Stichler (1978). This was a pilot study involving 105 women who were interviewed between the second and fourth post-operative days. Ninety-two per cent of the women reported feelings of fear about the surgery and anxiety and concern for themselves and the baby immediately prior to delivery; 52% reported dissatisfaction, anger or depression and 30% expressed feelings of relief that the labour was going to be terminated. In the survey 41% of the mothers expressed a need for reassurance, verbal communication or for touch prior to anaesthesia and explanations from professionals were the most commonly reported help in the preparation for section.

Another descriptive study was reported from Canada by Erb, Hill and Houston (1983). Women of mixed parity were self-selected through a media campaign and completed an open-ended questionnaire concerning their delivery experience. Of those women who had a primary (first) caesarean section, 93% expressed feelings of joy and relief alongside feelings of disappointment (68%), frustration (41%), failure (25%), guilt (20%) and anger (20%). These negative feelings were less pronounced if the women had previously experienced caesarean delivery.

Various other authors have reported similar negative responses to caesarean delivery. Studies by Cranley, Hedahl and Pegg (1983), Marut and Mercer (1979) and Trowell (1982) have suggested that feelings of guilt, failure, disappointment and anger are common among women delivered by section: a sense of failure at not being able to deliver the baby normally; a sense of guilt at putting the baby in danger and depriving her partner of the shared experience of birth and a sense of anger and disappointment at having been deprived of a normal birth herself.

From the published evidence available there appear to be several factors which to a limited extent may moderate some of these negative feelings. Among them, the most significant appear to be: the preparation for caesarean section; the type of anaesthesia employed and the presence of the father at delivery.

Preparation for caesarean section

Antenatal preparation classes should play an important role in preparing women for pregnancy, delivery and parenthood, however as in Chapter 8, Murphy-Black and Faulkner (1988) highlighted some of the criticisms of such classes which include poor preparation of sessions, conflicting advice and a lack of realism about the burdens of parenthood.

In Hillan's study (1992c), antenatal classes were criticised by 28% of the women and complaints occurred as frequently amongst women delivered vaginally as by caesarean section. The women felt that the teaching in these classes did not prepare them adequately for the experience of labour. Many women felt that the classes did not prepare them for any deviations from the course of normal labour such as slow progress or operative delivery. Explanations of caesarean section at classes were limited to elective deliveries for breech presentation and no mention was made of emergency sections during the course of labour. From some of the comments made by the women it appeared that in attempting to instil a positive attitude towards labour and delivery and the achievement of a spontaneous delivery, topics such as forceps delivery and caesarean section were downplayed or even ignored. During the year of the study in the hospital where the research was conducted, 15% of primigravidae had caesarean deliveries and a further 28% were delivered by forceps, so almost half had other than normal deliveries. As primigravidae are the main attenders at such classes and as it is impossible to predict which class members may require caesarean delivery before the onset of labour, it would seem appropriate that some discussion of alternative delivery methods should be included.

Type of anaesthesia

Another factor which may modify women's perceptions of their delivery experience is the type of anaesthesia employed for the operation. Available evidence suggests that women who have regional anaesthesia and are therefore able to remain conscious throughout, feel more in control of their situation and benefit from early parent–infant contact (Cranley, Hedahl and Pegg, 1983; Marut and Mercer, 1979). If general anaesthesia is used then it produces a gap in the woman's recollections and occasionally she may find it difficult to identify the infant as her own (Affonso, 1977). Hillan (1992c) noted that for some women delivered under general anaesthesia the sequence of events leading up to the decision to operate and immediately prior to the delivery was often confused. Clarifying the confusion and allowing the women the opportunity to reconstruct their experiences and express their feelings is an important and often neglected part of facilitating adjustment in the postnatal period. Midwives have an important role to play in counselling in this area. Although not all women can be given the choice or indeed want to be awake during surgery, if this is possible then women should have some choice in the type of anaesthesia used.

Presence of the father at delivery

The last major factor which appears to influence the psychosocial outcome of caesarean delivery is the presence of the father in the operating theatre. Various authors have shown that when partners were present, women expressed greater satisfaction with their delivery experience (Erb, Hill and Houston, 1983; Cranley, Hedahl and Pegg, 1983; Marut and Mercer, 1979). Fears about the adverse effects of the father's presence during surgery (such as the potential for increased infection, fathers fainting, lack of space and increased malpractice suits) have never been proved. Today both in the UK and the USA, a large number of hospitals allow fathers to be present in the operating theatre for delivery.

Maternal infant attachment

The performance of an emergency caesarean section will inevitably influence the amount of contact a mother has with her baby in the hour after delivery and in addition maternal reactions are likely to be affected by the stress associated with the operation. In a study of women delivered by emergency caesarean section, all had less than 90 minutes to prepare themselves for the operation and 80% knew of the decision for less than an hour before going to theatre. When told of the decision many of the women felt exhausted, frightened, confused or detached. Although 72% of the group saw the baby immediately at delivery, only 28% were actually allowed to hold the baby in theatre and this was usually just for a few moments before the baby was taken away. More than half of the women did not hold their baby in the 12 hours after delivery and 76% did not feed the baby in the 24-hour period following the birth. In contrast 90% of a vaginally delivered control group held the baby immediately and 92% had fed the infant within 24 hours. Seventy per cent of the women delivered vaginally were allowed some time alone with the baby and their partner after delivery although in over 70% of these cases the duration of such contact was less than half an hour (Hillan, 1992d).

Klaus and Kennel (1982) found some evidence that early mother–infant contact, especially during the first hour following delivery, is important though not critical for bonding. The promotion of bonding between the mother and her infant has become an increasingly important part of midwifery and obstetric care. The concept of bonding is characterized as being primarily unidirectional, occurring rapidly and facilitated by physical contact (Reading, 1983).

If regional anaesthesia is used, then the woman will be able, under normal circumstances, to enjoy seeing and holding her baby from the time that it is born and to share this experience with her partner. However, the woman delivered under general anaesthesia will have to wait until the effects of the anaesthetic have worn off before such contact can be enjoyed.

Marut and Mercer (1979) noted that in women delivered under general anaesthesia this process was delayed and that, in general, caesarean mothers' comments about their infants reflected hostility whereas vaginally delivered women's remarks primarily reflected concern.

In the light of these findings, it is probably not surprising that women in Hillan's (1992d) caesarian section group took longer than those in the control group to feel close to their infants. However, it must be remembered that:

> At present there are no definitive studies to either confirm or refute the existence of a sensitive period for bonding or to assess the length of time required in the first hours and days after birth to produce such an effect.
>
> Klaus and Kennel, 1983

Midwives are regarded as having an important role to play in ensuring that women have the opportunity to interact with their babies as soon as possible after delivery. However, further research is clearly needed in this field as it is difficult to assess the effects of caesarean delivery on the mother–infant relationship from the data already available. Most of the studies probably have a marked bias because of the sampling techniques employed and in any case, due to the differences in the health care systems between the USA and UK, would not necessarily be relevant in this country. Robson and Kumar (1980) showed that maternal affection may be lacking after any form of delivery and that this has been considered as a normal and even necessary variant, although Stichler and Affonso (1980) pointed out that the experiences which may facilitate bonding, such as early infant contact and rooming-in may be denied to women delivered by section. Unless there is a clear indication for observation in a special baby care unit, the routine admission of babies delivered by section to such units seems unnecessary.

Sexual adjustment following caesarean section

Hillan's study (1990) compared a group of primigravidae (first time mothers) delivered by caesarean section with a similar group of women delivered vaginally. One of the positive findings of this study was that women delivered by caesarean section resumed normal sexual relationships faster than women delivered vaginally and they also experienced fewer sexual problems after delivery. Six months after the birth of their babies, 14% of the women delivered vaginally were still experiencing what they considered serious sexual difficulties. For the majority of these women the major problem was due to perineal pain causing dyspareunia. In contrast, only 4% of women delivered by caesarean section complained of difficulties and these were caused by lack of interest due to tiredness.

Conclusions

Without doubt there is scope for further knowledge in this field which might go some way to improving the quality of caesarean childbirth for parents and also in preventing what Anne Oakley terms the 'psychosocial morbidity' associated with the 'new obstetrics'. There is at present insufficient knowledge of the efficacy, effectiveness and psychological impact of increasing caesarean section rates and comprehensive evaluative research is urgently needed to establish acceptable levels.

Further research is also required into the effects of the delivery method on mother–infant relations along with some determination of the adequacy of antenatal classes in meeting the needs of mothers who deliver by caesarean section.

Applications

1. Although not all women can be given the choice or indeed want to be awake during surgery, if this is possible then women should have some choice in the type of anaesthesia used.

2. In addition to the normal stressors associated with childbirth, women delivered by caesarean section have to cope with the aftermath of major surgery which may have occurred on top of a long and exhausting labour. Midwives and others should be aware of the need to promote the physical recovery of women in the immediate postnatal period.

3. For some women, particularly if delivered under general anaesthesia, the sequence of events leading up to the decision to operate and immediately prior to delivery may be confused. Clarifying this confusion and allowing women the opportunity to reconstruct their experiences is an important and often neglected part of facilitating adjustment in the postnatal period. Midwives have an important role to play in this area.

4. Women delivered by caesarean section may take longer to feel close to their infants than women delivered by other methods.

5. It is essential that staff involved in maternity care undertake systematic evaluation of the care given throughout the antenatal, intrapartum and postnatal period. Midwives are in direct contact with the women who use the maternity services. Therefore, they are ideally placed to ensure that perinatal audit develops into a much broader evaluation of the services, taking into account the views and opinions of consumers. The Changing Childbirth Report (HMSO, 1993) stresses the need for sound evidence to inform practice and highlights the importance of basing priorities for evaluation upon the expressed needs of women. Establishing priorities is a multifaceted process and may include both questions arising from clinical practice and those asked by care givers and by women and their families who use the services. Inevitably, such research will often be undertaken within a multidisciplinary context. Sleep (1995) suggests that the three criteria which should be used in determining priorities for future research are that the proposed research must meet the expressed needs of women, their babies and their families; offer the potential to improve the provision and standards of care; and be cost-effective in ensuring the most efficient use of service resources, research funding and research expertise.

Further reading

Francome, C., Savage, W., Churchill, H. and Lewison, H. (1993). *Caesarean Birth in Britain.* London: Middlesex University Press.
Enkin, M., Keirse, M., Renfrew, M. and Neilson, J. (1995). *A Guide to Effective Care in Pregnancy and Childbirth* (2nd ed). Oxford: Oxford University Press.

References

Affonso, D. (1977). Missing pieces: a study of post-partum feelings. *Birth and the Family Journal,* **4**, 159–64.
Affonso, D. and Stichler, J. (1978). Exploratory study of women's reactions to having a caesarean birth. *Birth and the Family Journal,* **5**, 88–94.
Affonso, D. and Stichler, J. (1980). Cesarean birth: women's reactions. *American Journal of Nursing,* **22**, 468–70.
Cranley, M. S., Hedahl, K. J. and Pegg, S. (1983). Women's perceptions of vaginal and ceasarean deliveries. *Nursing Research,* **32**, 10–15.
Erb, L., Hill, G. and Houston, D. (1983). A survey of parents' attitudes toward their cesarean births in Manitoba hospitals. *Birth,* **10**, 85–91.
Francome, C., Savage, W., Churchill, H. and Lewison, H. (1993). *Caesarean Birth in Britain.* London: Middlesex University Press.
Hall, M. H. (1995). Audit. In *The Future of the Maternity Services* (G. Chamberlain and N. Patel, eds). London: RCOG Press.
Hillan, E. M. (1990). Outcomes of Caesarean Section. University of Glasgow: Unpublished PhD thesis.
Hillan, E. M. (1992a). Short-term morbidity associated with cesarean delivery. *Birth,* **19**, 190–94.
Hillan, E. M. (1992b). Research and Audit: Women's Views of Caesarean Section. In *Women's Health Matters* (H. Roberts, ed.). London: Routledge.
Hillan, E. M. (1992c). Issues in the delivery of midwifery care. *Journal of Advanced Nursing,* **17** (1), 274–8.
Hillan, E. M. (1992d). Maternal-infant attachment following caesarean delivery. *Journal of Clinical Nursing,* **1**, 33–7.
HMSO (1993). Changing Childbirth – Report of the Export Maternity Group. London: HMSO.
Janis, I. L. (1958). *Psychological stress: psychoanalytic and behavioural studies of surgical patients.* New York: John Wiley and Sons.
Klaus, M. H., Jerauld, R., Kreger, B., McAlpine, W., Steffa, M. and Kennel, J. H. (1972). Maternal attachment. Importance of the first postpartum days. *New England Journal of Medicine,* **286**, 460–63.
Klaus, M. H. and Kennel, J. H. (1982). *Parent Infant Bonding.* St Louis: Mosby.
Kennel, J. H., Jerauld, R., Wolfe, H. et al. (1974). Maternal behaviour one year after early and extended postpartum contact. *Development Medicine and Child Neurology,* **16**, 172–9.
Marut, J. S. and Mercer, R. T. (1979). Comparison of primiparas' perceptions of vaginal and cesarean births. *Nursing Research,* **28**, 260–66.
Murphy-Black, T. and Faulkner, A. (1988). *Antenatal group skills training.* Edinburgh: John Wiley and Sons.
Oakley, A. (1980). *Women confined.* Oxford: Martin Robertson.
Oakley, A. (1983). Social consequences of obstetric technology: the importance of measuring 'soft' outcomes. *Birth,* **10**, 99–108.
O'Driscoll, K. and Foley, M. (1983). Correlation of decrease in perinatal mortality and increase in cesarean section rates. *Obstetrics and Gynecology,* **61**, 1–5.
Pearson, J. W. (1984). Caesarean section and perinatal mortality. *American Journal of Obstetrics and Gynecology,* **148**, 155–9.

Reading, A. J. (1983). 'Bonding'. In *Progress in Obstetrics and Gynaecology*, Vol. III (J. Studd, ed.). Edinburgh: Churchill Livingstone.

Robson, K. M. and Kumar, R. (1980). Delayed onset of maternal affection after childbirth. *British Journal of Psychistry*, **136**, 347–53.

Rosen, M. G. (1981). Cesarean Childbirth: report of a consensus development conference. Bethesda, Maryland: National Institute of Health (NIH Publication no. 82-2067).

Shearer, M. H. (1983). The difficulty of measuring satisfaction with perinatal care. *Birth*, **10**, 77.

Sleep, J. (1995). Areas of future research in the maternity services. In *The Future of the Maternity Services* (G. Chamberlain and N. Patel, eds). London: RCOG Press.

Stichler, J. and Affonso, D. (1980). Cesarean birth. *American Journal of Nursing*, March, 466–8.

Thiery, M. and Derom, R. (1986). Review of evaluative studies on caesarean section. Part I: Trends in caesarean section and perinatal mortality. In *Perinatal care delivery systems* (M. Kamininiski, B. Gerard, P. Buekins, H. J. Huisjes, G. McIlwaine, H. K. Selbman, eds). Oxford: Oxford University press.

Trowell, J. (1982). Possible effects of emergency caesarean section on the mother child relationship. *Early Human Development*, **7**, 41–51.

11

Perinatal pain

Catherine Niven and Karel Gijsbers

> In this chapter Catherine Niven and Karel Gijsbers discuss some of the central
> puzzles of labour pain: why is it so painful; why does it vary so much; why does it
> exist at all? In addition they show that labour pain is only one of a range of pains
> with which women cope in the process of reproducing, and suggest that the
> physiological and psychological aspects of these experiences may interact.
>
> This chapter should be read in conjunction with Chapter 8 which deals with
> preparation for childbirth and Chapter 9 on birth experiences.

Texts which consider pain in the perinatal period traditionally focus on labour
pain to the exclusion of other pain experiences. We will argue that although
labour pain is on average more intense than other reproductive pain experiences,
it is not the only pain associated with giving birth. Perinatal pain may be best
regarded as a continuum over time which varies in nature and intensity and in its
associations with various aspects of the reproductive process – pregnancy,
labour, delivery, postnatal recovery, breast feeding.

Perinatal pain experiences

Pregnancy is more often characterized by discomfort than by pain but
prospective studies have shown that back ache and severe leg cramps are also
common (Wolkind and Zajicek, 1981). In contrast, birth is certainly characterized by pain but also by the most positive of life events – new life. As we
discuss below, childbirth can involve the most intense pain a woman will
experience in her lifetime and typically involves severe pain at some point
during the process of labour and delivery, although pain levels vary considerably.
Severe, prolonged, unrelieved pain in labour can result in maternal and fetal
stress (Bonica, 1984; Stewart, 1982).

During the postnatal period women may experience uterine cramps, perineal
pain and nipple pain. Uterine cramps or 'after-pains' which are caused by the
contraction of the uterus after delivery, occur intermittently for about five days
postnatally, especially in multiparous women where the uterus is more bulky.
Pain levels average around 60 on a 1–100 visual analogue scale, with 50–75%
of women who experience cramps complaining of 'severe pain' (Skovlund,
Fyllingen, Landre and Neshcim, 1991). Uterine cramping is commonly
associated with breast feeding and peaks at the same time as nipple pain, making
the early experience of breast feeding a painful one for many mothers. The
incidence of nipple pain declines from around 60% of breast feeding mothers
on the second postpartum day to 20–25% on both the fifteenth and thirtieth day
(Drewett, Kahn, Parkhurst and Whiteley, 1987).

On the first postnatal day, mild perineal pain affects around 50% of women
who have an intact perineum. This compares with around 80% of women who

have suffered a spontaneous tear in their perineum during delivery, who suffer mild or moderate pain, and more than 95% of women who have had a episiotomy (the surgical enlargement of the vaginal orifice carried out during delivery), 30% of whom experience severe pain (Larsson, Platz-Christensen, Bergman and Wallstersson, 1991). Fifteen to thirty-seven per cent still complain of pain on the third postnatal day (Thacker and Banta, 1983) and 10% at three months (Reading, 1982). Dysparunia (painful sexual intercourse) is reported by around 80% of women who have had episiotomies compared to 60% of women who had lacerations with rates at three months of 19% and at 12 months, 8% (Reading, 1982; Robson and Kumar, 1981).

Pain in women

Strictly speaking, perinatal pain is pain occurring in the few months immediately preceding and following birth. But pain in pregnancy, birth and the postnatal period should not be viewed in isolation from other pains which a woman can experience. Back pain suffered in the later part of pregnancy is related to the level of subsequent labour pain, but so is the level of menstrual pain suffered before pregnancy (Melzack and Belanger, 1989). Explanations of these relationships are not straightforward but could depend on factors such as the size of the baby and levels of the prostaglandin hormone. The size of the baby would affect the load on the back muscles during pregnancy and pressure on the cervix and walls of the birth canal during delivery, while prostaglandin levels affect the strength of uterine contraction both during menstruation and childbirth.

These data emphasize that pains outwith labour are directly related to those experienced during childbirth. This relationship is not necessarily only of a physiological nature; changes in psychological attitudes could also be involved. There is experimental evidence that the experience of labour pain affects the way in which women react to other types of pain not related to childbirth. For example, the threshold to pain induced systematically by immersion of an arm in cold water has been reported to be higher in women who have given birth when compared with that of nulliparous women (Hapidou and DeCatanzaro, 1992). These differences can be understood in terms of labour pain providing a benchmark for assessing other forms of pain. And it is reasonable to expect other reciprocal psychological relationships between the perception of labour pain and general pain experiences. In particular, the regular experience of menstrual pain could provide an opportunity for women to develop coping strategies that can be transferred to the childbirth situation (Niven and Gijsbers, 1984, in press).

Many women experience pain in the pelvis outwith pregnancy and the postpartum period. While some of these pains are pathological in origin, relating to problems of the endometrium (lining of the uterus), venous perfusion of pelvic structure or infection of fallopian tubes, healthy women regularly experience extensive episodes of 'normal' pain arising from abdominal viscera, such as dysmenorrhea, the pain associated with menstruation. Regular experiences of visceral pain may have constitutional consequences relating to the physiological mechanisms mediating pain responses. The commonsense point of view is that pain is produced by tissue-damaging ('noxious') stimulation activating specific sensory receptors and nerve fibres that respond to high-intensity sensory input. Such systems exist throughout the body, but clinical evidence indicates that in some circumstances pain can be provoked by stimuli that are not normally thought to be noxious in nature. Neurophysiological research has shown that elements of the nervous system that normally respond to non-noxious stimuli can, after a period of continuous pain, become involved in exciting cells in the central nervous system that would normally only be activated by stimuli in the painful range. In addition, there exists what have been termed 'silent nociceptors', receptor systems that are capable of signalling pain but which are normally inactive. These switch in after an extended period of pain, thus additionally contributing to an overly sensitized nervous system. The implication for women who regularly suffer episodes of visceral pain is that they might possess a sensitized visceral pain system. This hypothesis has been used to explain Irritable Bowel Syndrome (Cervero, 1994). Whether sensitization occurs more generally to other pains of a visceral nature is of course speculative. But the possibility exists that women can become predisposed to experience visceral pain such as that involved in menstruation and childbirth.

During pregnancy however, the situation may be different. Research in animals has shown a decreased sensitivity to pain over the course of pregnancy, most notably immediately prior to parturition (birth). This effect appears to be mediated by endorphins, the morphine-like substances found in mammalian brains (Gintzler, 1980). These data support the supposition that endorphins provide a 'natural antidote' or 'analgesic' for pain during childbirth and that their pain-reducing effects would be evident in the latter stages of pregnancy. However, the evidence for this supposition in human studies is not conclusive. It has been reported that pain sensitivity to mechanical pressure on the arm is reduced during the last few days of pregnancy (Cogan and Spinnato, 1986) but other studies using human subjects found either no changes in pain sensitivity during late pregnancy, labour and post delivery or an increase in pain sensitivity during pregnancy (Dunbar, Price and Newton, 1988; Goolkasian and Rimer, 1984).

It needs to be recognized that estimating endorphin levels in the brain and spinal cord during pregnancy and labour is by no means simple. In fact, most studies of endorphin levels in pregnant women have based their estimates on venous blood samples which have no direct relationship with levels in the central nervous systems. Whether endorphins actually increase in the brain during pregnancy and labour in a way consistent with a decrease in pain sensitivity is thus open to question (Eisenach, Dobson, Inturrisi et al., 1990). Furthermore, actual levels of endorphins in the brain may not be as important in determining perceived levels of pain intensity as the degree of sensitivity of brain cells to endorphins which would be extremely difficult to assess in the brains of living human females.

It is possible that the style of testing is a significant factor in revealing changes in pain sensitivity during pregnancy. In addition, in human subjects, anxiety and apprehension concerning the imminent labour experience may play a role that is absent in non-human animals. This apprehension might counteract any positive analgesic effects of increased endorphin levels.

Female rats also show decreased sensitivity to noxious stimulation during vaginal probing that mimics the pressure on the vaginal wall and cervix that occurs during copulation and parturition. These effects are mediated by inter-actions between nerve fibres serving the vagina and cervix, female sex hormones and noradrenalin and seratonin neurotransmitters (Steinman, Komisaruk, Yaksh and Tyce, 1983). Preliminary studies by Whipple and Komisaruk (1985) with human female subjects have demonstrated similar changes in pain sensitivity during vaginal stimulation. The same research group has also reported increases in pain threshold to tactile stimulation to the fingers during childbirth, again with no change in non-painful tactile threshold. This only occurred for subjects who had undergone Lamaze-type preparation for birth. In fact, subjects without child-birth preparation showed an increased sensitivity to experimentally-induced pain during labour (Whipple, Josimovich and Komisaruk, 1990). A possible explanation for these conflicting data is that the analgesia produced by the peripheral physiological mechanisms can be moderated by psychological factors such as anxiety and stress.

It should be emphasized that this work, while very intriguing, needs to be sub-stantiated. However both sets of studies, those focusing on endorphin production during pregnancy, and those on monoamines released by stimulation of the vagina, suggest that while women may be predisposed to be particularly sensitive to visceral pain, pain during birth may be mitigated by neural mechanisms relating to reproduction. For the human female, these mechanisms operate in some form of balance with psychological attitudes generated by gender-based experiences of pain.

Labour pain

Childbirth is a complex biological, social and psychological event which takes place in several stages. The first stage of labour consists of the dilation of the cervix from the pre-labour stage of nondilation to the maximal dilation of 10 cm. This involves the co-ordinated contraction of the uterine muscles which occur at intervals. Contractions become more frequent as labour progresses to a maximum frequency of about 2–3 every 10 minutes. The time taken to achieve full cervical dilation varies considerably, lasting 8–12 hours on average in primiparous women (women giving birth for the first time) and less in subsequent deliveries. The second stage of labour begins when complete cervical dilation is achieved and ends when the baby is delivered. During delivery, the conscious efforts of the mother to bear down amplify the intrinsic explosive mechanisms. In the normal labour where the head is the presenting part and where the pelvis is adequately shaped, the baby's head descends into the mid-pelvis, rotates, moves downwards distending the vulva and appears at the exterior – 'crowning'. The shoulders and then the head turns and the baby is delivered. This birth process generally takes about 50 minutes in a primiparous woman and 20 minutes if she is multiparous (having her second or subsequent child). The third stage of labour involves the delivery of the placenta and is usually achieved in a few contractions.

Thus childbirth is a lengthy, dynamic process, the efficiency of which is determined by complex and changing interactions between uterine muscle contraction, the resistance of the cervix and other pelvic structures, and the 'fit' between the size and shape of the birth canal and the size, shape and orientation of the baby.

The intensity of labour pain

The vast majority of studies which have attempted to quantify the intensity of labour pain have been carried out in developed countries where childbirth is a medicalized event and most births take place in hospital with trained medical or midwifery staff in attendance, e.g. Sweden (Fridth, Kopare, Gaston-Johansson and Norvell, 1988); the USA (Lowe, 1989); Canada (Melzack, 1984); Australia (Astbury, 1980); England (Scott-Palmer and Skevington, 1981); Scotland (Niven and Gijsbers, 1984) and Kuwait (Harrison, 1991). Such studies vary in their methodology with labour pain being assessed on numerical, semantic and visual analogue scales. The timing of its assessment can also vary with the majority of studies assessing first-stage labour while others, despite the practical and ethical difficulties involved assess delivery. Since labour pain usually increases from early labour, to late first-stage labour, to crowning, the timing of labour pain assessment will affect comparability across studies (Scott-Palmer and Skevington, 1981). Timing effects may be compounded by subject charac-teristics such as parity (Gaston-Johansson, Fridth and Turner-Norvell, 1988). Furthermore, a number of labour pain studies utilize retrospective measures. Since it is difficult for subjects to isolate recall of pain at one particular point in time, e.g. delivery, it is likely that retrospective pain assessment taps the recollection of labour at its most painful or some cumulative measure of the pain of repeated contractions. Although retrospective assessment has been criticized because of the possible confounding effects of memory and mood (Norvell, Gaston-Johansson and Fridth, 1988), it does offer an overview of the woman's experience of many hours of intermittent pain which cross-sectional assessments cannot access.

The intensity of labour pain will obviously be affected by the use of analgesia. Women in labour routinely receive analgesic drugs and/or treatments such as TENS (transcutaneous electrical nerve stimulation) which are designed to reduce levels of pain. Labour pain management techniques vary in their potential effectiveness. Lumbar epidural anaesthesia, which involves the introduction of a local anaesthetic injection into the epidural space of the lumbar section of the spinal cord, thereby blocking sensory impulses from the uterus, cervix and perineum can produce total analgesia (Crawford, 1972). Analgesics like pethidine (Demerol) which is injected or nitrous oxide in oxygen (Entonox) which is inhaled, usually reduce pain rather than abolishing it. Therefore it might be expected that labour pain levels would normally be low. However, medical concerns about the effects that analgesics might have in inhibiting progress in labour and on the condition of the baby have led to obstetric policies which restrict the use of analgesia. Epidural anaesthesia is often only commenced once labour is well established, when pain levels are already high (Melzack, 1984); potent analgesic drugs such as pethidine are only given in relatively small amounts and not close to delivery (Bonica, 1975) and the availability of Entonox is sometimes restricted by midwifery staff to later in labour (Niven and Gijsbers, 1984). Furthermore, mothers-to-be often plan to use little or no analgesia in labour in an effort to ensure 'natural' childbirth. Although a substantial pro-portion of these women subsequently change their mind, they only do so after having experienced considerable pain (Melzack, 1984; Niven and Gijbers, 1984). Thus the potential for labour pain reduction is often not fulfilled, despite the availability of a variety of analgesic drugs and treatments. This has clear clinical implications which are discussed at the end of this chapter. However, in methodological terms, it does reduce the effects of one potentially potent source of variability in labour pain levels.

Given the difficulties inherent in the study of labour pain, remarkable congruence between studies is apparent, with labour pain on average being assessed as very intense. Studies which have used the same methodology, such as those carried out by Melzack and colleagues in a large city hospital in Canada (Melzack, Taenzer, Feldman and Kinch, 1981) and by Niven and Gijsbers (1984) in a small town hospital in Scotland show substantial agreement on pain intensity. Both studies used the McGill Pain Questionnaire (MPQ) (Melzack, 1975) to assess the intensity and quality of labour pain. Results not only found that levels of labour pain were amongst the most intense every measured by the MPQ but also showed substantial agreement on pain quality, labour pain being described as 'stabbing'. 'sharp', 'cramping', 'exhausting' and 'penetrating' by more than 50% of subjects in both studies.

Despite the stress inherent in childbirth and the intense pain that most women experience, the pain of childbirth is not typically described as being intensely negative in affect. Studies carried out in western hospitals show that descriptors such as 'terrifying', 'cruel' and 'wretched' are infrequently selected to describe labour pain (Melzack, Taenzer, Feldman and Kinch, 1981; Niven and Gijsbers, 1984; Gaston-Johansson, Fridth and Turner-Norvell, 1988). This contrasts with other types of severe pain such as toothache or cancer which typically have a high affective component (Melzack, 1975) and presumably reflects the different meaning of these pains; labour pain being unusual in its positive connotations. However, it should be noted that a proportion of women giving birth do describe labour pain in strongly negative terms. It may be more important to ameliorate these negative aspects of labour pain than to reduce the intensity of labour pain overall (Niven, 1986; Harrison, 1991).

Advocates of 'home birth' have challenged the findings that show labour pain to be intense, suggesting that births which take place in familiar, non-medicalized settings are normally less painful (e.g. Kitzinger, 1989). Unfortunately properly controlled studies have not been carried out comparing pain levels in home births with those in hospital births. Data on labour pain in 'non-developed' societies is extremely scarce though a study of childbirth in Fiji, where women normally give birth using traditional practices, found that Fijian women rated labour pain as severe, being ranked as considerably more painful than the pain of a broken leg or toothache (Morse, 1989). The myth that women in less advanced technological/medicalized societies give birth with little fuss and pain, delivering their babies and immediately recommencing their work in the fields has not been substantiated. Ethnographic studies suggest instead that all properly functioning societies (i.e. those which are not at war or in decline due to cultural pollution, famine, etc.) place great emphasis on specialized treatment of the woman giving birth, with herbal preparations, massage and body mechanics being used to relieve pain (Cosminsky, 1977). Thus data from a number of cultures obtained through the use of diverse methodology suggests that childbirth is normally painful.

Notwithstanding this evidence, early and continuing theoretical debate has centred on the question of why labour pain exists at all. Pain after all is usually associated with tissue damage, disease or functional disorder whereas childbirth is part of normal female physiological functioning. Labour pain also appears to be unique to the human species of primate (Rushton and McGrew, 1989; Linburg, 1982) but see Gijsbers and McGrew (1985). These considerations, have led some people to expect that humans should, and could, have similarly pain-free 'natural' labours, arguing that 'there is no physiological function in the body which gives rise to pain in the normal course of health' Dick Read (1947) (an argument which ignores the evidence of pain associated with normal menstruation). However, in humans the pelvic girdle to fetal head ratio is such that there is a much 'tighter fit' than is the case in non-human primates (Linburg, 1982). This is due to the evolutionary development of the large human cerebral cortex, giving a large fetal head, and to the reduction in the dimensions of the birth canal associated with bipedal gait. Consequently birth in humans is more likely to invoke potentially painful stimuli.

Pain which occurs during the first stage of labour is generally thought to result from the dilation of the cervix and contraction of the uterus. Dilation of the cervix in pregnant and in non-pregnant women produces pain similar in quality and spatial distribution to that produced during labour, the more rapid the dilation (induced artificially by means of inflating a small balloon inserted into the cervix) the more intense the pain (Bonica and Akamatsu, 1975). Uterine contractions do not typically become painful until 15 to 20 seconds after their onset, the amount of time needed for the contraction to distend the lower uterus and cervix (Bonica, 1975). However, while labour pain is generally expected to be felt in the abdomen and to be intermittent, coinciding with the contractions of the uterus, Melzack and colleagues (1991) have clearly demonstrated that the timing and distribution of pain is more variable, with back pain being almost as common as abdominal pain and approximately one third of subjects experiencing continuous pain as well as contraction pain. The release of pain-inducing prostaglandins may sensitize pain receptors during labour (see above) and add additional sources of noxious (potentially pain-producing) stimulation at that time as the distention and superficial traumatization of the vagina and perineum, traction and pressure on pelvic nerves, organs and fascia do during delivery.

Thus there are a number of sources of noxious stimulation in childbirth which are transmitted from the cervix and uterus via sensory (pain) fibres to the spinal cord. (It is these transmission pathways which are blocked by regional anaesthesia.)

Labour pain variability

Although labour pain is on average intense, individual levels of labour pain vary widely. For example a study of labour pain in over 100 healthy Scottish women found pain levels in the active phase of the first stage of labour varying from 0 to 9.5 on a 10 cm visual analogue scale and recall of labour and delivery pain levels ranging from 1.5 to 10 (Niven and Gijsbers, 1984). Thus any theory which attempts to explain labour pain needs to address not only why it is, on average, so intense but also why it varies so much.

Variability in labour pain may be simply explained by variation in the bio-dynamics of the birth process with a physically efficient labour involving less noxious stimulation and therefore less pain than an inefficient one. As early as 1933 however, Dick Read was hypothesizing that some of the variation occurring in the perception of pain in childbirth was due to psychological factors.

Specifically he claimed that high levels of anxiety were the cause of intense labour pain (Dick Read, 1933, 1947). The then current model of pain transmission only allowed him to explain this contentious supposition by means of inferring an accompanying increase in noxious stimulation. He hypothesized that increased anxiety led to contraction of the cervix through the actions of the sympathetic nervous system. The pressure of the baby's head being forced down on to the contracted cervix during uterine contractions produced high levels of noxious stimulation and hence high levels of labour pain (Dick Read, 1947). It is now known that the cervix contains very little contractile tissue and is more likely to be dilating than contracting during periods of maximal labour pain (Bonica, 1975; Bonica and Akamatsu, 1975). Therefore Dick Read's hypothesis concerning the mechanisms of labour pain transmission in conditions of high maternal anxiety has been brought into question. However, many reviewers have concluded that variation in physiological factors is insufficient to explain the extreme variability which characterizes labour pain, e.g. Bonica (1975). Accordingly, variability has been attributed in part to psychological factors.

Empirical studies have associated variability in labour pain with a huge number of factors. For example, higher levels of labour pain have been generally found to be associated with factors as diverse as primiparity (first birth), age, lower socio-economic status, unrealistic expectations of pain, artificial rupture of the membranes (a technique used to induce labour), higher maternal weight/height ratio and as discussed above, the previous experience of menstrual pain or menstrual difficulties. Lower levels of pain have been associated with delivery at night, confidence in the ability to handle labour pain, attendance at classes which aim to prepare women for childbirth and the use, and previous experience of using, certain pain coping strategies (see Fridth, Kopare and Gaston-Johansson, 1988; Lowe, 1989; Marx, 1979; Melzack, 1984; Niven, 1986; Niven and Gijsbers, 1984; Harrison, 1991; Harkness and Gijsbers, 1989). However, research studies have not always confirmed these findings (e.g. Copstick, Taylor, Hayes and Morris, 1986; Niven, 1986) and variables related to personality or the presence of the husband at birth have been associated with both significant increases *and* decreases in levels of labour pain in different studies (see Niven, 1992 for review). Thus while no definitive list of factors affecting labour pain can yet be constructed, research has shown that labour pain is subject to bio-psycho-social modulation.

Methodological differences in subject selection and pain assessment abound in labour pain research and practical and ethical constraints have led to a plethora of studies with small numbers, inadequate control groups, and a lack of empirical rigour. This may explain the heterogeneity of findings. The very complexity of the physical and psychological aspects of childbirth and the interactions between them may also account for differences between studies. However, real differences in attitudes to childbirth, labour pain and labour pain behaviour are apparent across cultures. Together with differences in the ways that childbirth is managed between countries and between and within hospitals, these differences may account for some of the variability in research results on factors affecting labour pain. For instance, a major cross-cultural study showed that attitudes towards labour pain varied extensively between the Yucatan, Holland, Sweden and the USA (Jordan, 1980). These attitudes were reflected in birthing systems which highlighted or discounted pain or which served to make childbirth visible or invisible and viewed as either a medical or natural event. A more recent study of two distinct cultural groups within Fiji makes the same point, with Fijian society emphasizing the community aspects of health, including birth which takes place within sound but not sight of the community including the men. Women assist at the delivery, their role being to soothe the mother. Labour is regarded as a severely painful experience but labour pain should be tolerated. In contrast, in Fiji-Indian society, female innocence and purity are valued highly. The sexual aspects of childbirth are therefore a source of shame and embarrassment and pregnancy is kept a secret for as long as possible and not discussed within the community. Birth is a hidden event except from the midwife. Labour pain is devalued especially by the males (Morse, 1989).

These examples of cultural differences are clear cut but more subtle differences between cultures are also likely to have effects on attitudes to childbirth and labour pain. One might compare the attitude of a catholic mother of five giving birth in a maternity home run by nuns where she is told to 'offer your pain up for the Holy souls in Purgatory' (personal communication) with those of a first-time mother who has followed the advice given in a recent publication '(during labour) Mother earth will be there to support, nourish and sustain you. ... There will be a constant exchange between your body and the ground, where the earth absorbs the pain and gives back new, fresh energy' (Balaskas, 1994). These mothers come from the same overall culture, that of the UK, but their attitudes are likely to be quite distinct.

Differences in attitude to childbirth and its associated pain can also be seen between classes. Working-class women in the UK and US have been shown to place little value on the experience of childbirth per se. Labour is merely something which has to be gone through in order to have a baby. The concern about childbirth is that it is as quick and safe as possible, involves the minimum of pain and allows the woman to maintain her dignity. Middle-class women on the other hand have been shown to more frequently focus on the nature of the experience of childbirth in its own right as one which holds a potential for pleasure and reward. A desire for a 'natural' childbirth with a minimum of intervention and analgesia is more apparent in middle-class women (Nelson, 1983; McIntosh, 1989). Such differences in attitude to childbirth and to labour pain interact with obstetric policy and can have profound effects on the experience of labour pain. At extremes such effects can produce, on the one hand, a relatively painless labour for a woman who wishes to have a pain-free labour in a hospital which provides an epidural service available to all, or a pain-filled labour for a woman having a difficult birth who seeks a 'natural childbirth' without analgesics, or has one imposed upon her because analgesics are not available. More subtle interactions between attitudes to childbirth, attitudes to pain and obstetric management regimens may also have an effect on labour pain levels which is less apparent and therefore less easy to control empirically or statistically.

Furthermore, childbirth normally takes place in a social setting and some research suggests that the social interactions between the mother and her birth attendants have a powerful effect on her experience of childbirth (Kennel, Klaus, McGrath, 1988; Niven, 1994). Thus more emphasis on the study of interactions between key individuals during labour might clarify some of the confusion which surrounds the study of factors affecting labour pain variability. The effect of social interactions may be dependent on social support mechanisms acting either directly or indirectly on the stress which is intrinsic to giving birth. One source of this stress is labour pain, which can evoke intense fear and anxiety. This, in turn, can exacerbate levels of pain, leading to a spiralling pain/stress-circle (Melzack and Wall, 1993). The amelioration of stress in childbirth through social support (Folkman, 1984) may thus ameliorate labour pain.

Thus far we have suggested that the reasons for individual differences in levels of childbirth pain may be mechanical (to do with the 'goodness of fit' between the fetus and the birth canal); obstetric (related to the medical/midwifery regimen); psychological or social. An alternative physiological view might attribute them to differences in peripheral visceral sensitization as discussed earlier in this chapter, or individual differences in levels of endorphins or in the hormones that prepare the internal reproductive organs for childbirth. Some support for this idea is given by the observation that women who give birth at night, as do most primates, report having less pain than those that give birth during the day (Harkness and Gijbers, 1989) when, presumably, the complex hormonal synchronization supporting birth may not be at its optimum. Women who suffer little pain while giving birth also claim to have experienced little or no pain outwith labour (Niven and Gijbers, 1989) suggesting that there is some pervading difference in their pain mechanisms.

Currently, there is no evidence that correlates individual levels of labour pain to any specific physiological mechanism. However, modern theories of pain such as 'Gate control' theory proposed by Melzack and Wall (1993), envisage the processing of information related to pain perception, even at its earliest stages, as being crucially influenced by psychological factors related to emotion and cognition. Subsequent research has identified a number of structures deep in the brain that not only receive information concerning pain from the spinal cord, but in turn project down onto those cells in the spinal cord that are involved in pain responses. An accessible review is given in Melzack and Wall (1993).

One such structure deep in the core of the brain or brainstem, is called the Periaqueductal Gray (PAG). Direct electrical stimulation of the PAG produces profound analgesia (Hosobuchi, Adams and Linchitz, 1977). This is mediated by inhibitory pathways to the spinal cord that involve both the endorphins and monoamine brain chemicals. The PAG also receives inputs from structures further upstream in the brain, including the hypothalamus which is involved in motivational processes, the limbic system which is involved in emotional changes, and frontal areas implicated in complex cognitive activity. Thus it can be seen that the PAG, a structure that has a dominant influence on pain processing at its earliest stages, is in turn influenced by a broad range of brain structures implicated in high order psychological processes. Consequently, in view of what we know about the physiological mechanisms mediating pain it would be surprising if no variability was found in reports of levels of pain from human females, even during normal healthy births. It is to be expected that women approaching labour vary considerably in their emotional states, expectancies, memories and competence to deal with pain and stress. This variability will find expression in the physiological control processes that are intrinsic to the transmission of information concerning pain, resulting in considerable variability in levels of consciously perceived pain.

Conclusions

Pain certainly abounds in the perinatal period. Childbirth commonly, but not invariably, involves severe pain, and the postnatal period can be dominated not by rest and recovery but by nipple pain, perineal pain and uterine cramps. However, as we have discussed in this chapter, women are used to pain and are frequently skilled in coping with its manifestations. Perhaps because of this, labour pain, while on average intense, is not often experienced as intensely aversive. Indeed, some women consider that pain is a desirable part of childbirth (Purdie, Reid, Thorburn and Asbury, 1992; Curry, Pascoo and Heap, 1994). Physiologically however, the experience of severe pain may be undesirable as it is associated with reflex increases in blood pressure and oxygen consumption which can be harmful to the fetus during childbirth and may, if prolonged, lead to sensitization of the central nervous system. Many women wish to reduce or abolish perinatal pain, a completely logical desire which is unfortunately not always fulfilled despite the huge range of analgesic drugs, treatments and techniques potentially available. In the Applications section below we discuss how perinatal pain relief may be better achieved.

Modern theories of pain are psycho-physiological and thus offer a better framework for the consideration of perinatal pain than theories which look at physiological or psychological aspects of pain in isolation. Pain in childbirth is however additionally influenced by the biomechanics of the birth process, involving two individuals – the mother and the fetus – not just one, and along with other forms of perinatal pain is set in a medical and social context. The theoretical, empirical and clinical challenge for the future is to incorporate all these components in a bio-psycho-social framework for perinatal pain.

Applications

Just as research on perinatal pain experience has been dominated by labour pain, so the consideration of its amelioration has been focused unduly on labour pain. This focus has led to the relative neglect of other perinatal pain experiences such as perinatal pain or nipple pain. Research on labour pain amelioration has been inconclusive, since large numbers of drugs (from heroin to sterile water) and techniques (from transcutaneous nerve stimulation to music-assisted birth) have been used in an as yet unsuccessful attempt to find one which can be made widely available, is acceptable to all mothers, safe for both mother and baby and is reliably effective in reducing or abolishing labour pain.

The use of epidural anaesthesia has been the major advance in obstetric anaesthesiology in recent years. It can, when successful, allow the mother to have a pain-free labour. However, in unskilled hands it can fail to produce satisfactory pain relief in up to 33% of cases (Melzack, 1984) and its use has been associated with side-effects and is sometimes unpopular (MacArthur, Lewis and Knox, 1992; Morgan, Bulpitt, Clifton and Lewis 1982).

Knowledge about pain reduction has increased massively in recent decades informed by the modern psycho-physiological theories of pain. Thus pain-reduction techniques, even when primarily physiological or pharmacological, take into consideration the psychological aspects of treatment and psychological analgesia is no longer regarded as the perogative of alternative medicine but instead as a form of complementary therapy which can supplement, as well as replace, pharmacological analgesics. The modern approach to pain reduction, applied to the consideration of perinatal pain would suggest that:

1. The source of pain is avoided if possible

Common sense suggests that if we can avoid a potential cause of pain, we should. Theories of pain transmission also suggest that the experience of pain may sensitize the central nervous system (see above). Many sources of perinatal pain such as labour pain cannot be avoided but some which are associated with routine intervention or practice can be obviated, at least partially. For example, since the necessity for routine episiotomy has been challenged, rates of episiotomy have fallen dramatically, sparing many women the experience of episiotomy-related perineal pain (Thacker and Banta, 1983; Larsson, Platz-Christensen, Bergman and Wallstersson, 1991). Similarly, nipple pain is associated with rigid breast feeding regimens, so feeding on demand reduces its likelihood (Illingworth and Stone, 1952).

2. Analgesic drugs, if used, are given before pain becomes intense

Traditional pharmacological approaches to pain relief have involved the provision of analgesics in response to pain. Research has clearly demonstrated that this is an inefficient treatment regimen and that smaller amounts of analgesics produce better control of pain if they are used to prevent intense pain, not respond to it (American Pain Society, 1989). Thus in labour, consideration should be given to ameliorating labour pain *before* it becomes intense provided that early administration does not have a negative effect on progress in labour. This would have the additional benefit of reducing stress and anxiety, thus preventing the harmful effects of stress on the fetus as well as the mother and short-circuiting the vicious pain–stress circle. In the postnatal period, all women who have perineal damage could be encouraged to take analgesics to prevent the experience of perineal pain.

3. Analgesic drugs, if used, are 'parturant-controlled'

The issue of who controls the use of analgesics has been central to both political and psychological issues in pain relief for some time and has led to the widespread use of patient-controlled analgesia (PCA). This technique involves the patient having control over the timing and frequency of use of potent analgesic drugs administered by injection or through the epidural route. The maximum dose which can be administered is set but otherwise the patient self-administers the drug by pressing a button on the PCA apparatus. This technique has only recently come into use in obstetrics where the anaesthetist initially establishes satisfactory epidural anaesthesia and the parturant subsequently administers 'top-up' doses. Early studies indicate its use in obstetrics is as successful as it has been in cancer pain control and post-operatively, where it has been found to yield high levels of patient satisfaction combined with efficient, effective analgesia (Curry, Pascoo and Heap, 1994; Paech, 1992; Purdie, Reid, Thorburn and Astbury, 1992).

Patient-controlled epidural anaesthesia is not universally available since it necessitates fairly sophisticated technology along with the presence of an experienced anaesthetist. The broad principles of PCA could be usefully extended to less sophisticated analgesic methods. The use of Entonox which involves very simple technology and is widely available, is one such method. The amount and timing of its administration is directly under the control of the parturant and so may have many of the psychological benefits offered by PCA.

4. Accurate information on labour pain, if requested, is made available

Research concerned with reactions to stressful or painful medical experiences such as surgery has demonstrated that the provision of preparatory information can improve outcome especially when that information is accurate, involves detailed description of the sensations likely to be experienced ('sensory information') and includes coping information, e.g. Johnson, Rice, Fullar and Endress (1978). This type of information encourages the subject to normalize their experience and facilitates coping. The use of sensory information could be emphasized in preparation for childbirth so as to make the anticipated experience more realistic and facilitate coping (see Niven, 1992, for a detailed discussion).

5. Psychological analgesia is made more effective

As Niven has argued elsewhere (Niven, 1992) antenatal training should be complemented by intranatal training in techniques of pain reduction so that women in early labour would have directly relevant, personalized training in the use of psychological analgesia, the effectiveness of which would be thus immediately apparent, boosting their confidence in coping with pain throughout labour and delivery. The use of psychological analgesia could be encouraged in the pre- and postnatal periods as an alternative or complement to the use of analgesic drugs.

6. Perinatal pain is related to the woman's general experience of pain

A woman's ability to cope with labour pain and the pains of the postnatal period can be enhanced through reference to her general pain experience. By encouraging a woman to use familiar, successful coping strategies, antenatal or intranatal educators can increase the range of strategies available to the woman in labour and enhance her sense of self-efficacy.

Further reading

Gijsbers, K. and Niven, C. A. (1993). Women and the experience of pain. In *The Health Psychology of Women* (C. A. Niven and D. Carroll, eds). Switzerland: Harwood Academic Publishers.

Melzack, R. (1984). The myth of painless childbirth. *Pain*, 19, 321–7.

Melzack, R. and Wall, P. (1993). *The Challenge of Pain*. Harmondsworth: Penguin.

References

American Pain Society (1989). *Principles of Analgesic Use in the Treatment of Acute Pain and Chronic Cancer Pain*. Illinois: American Pain Society.

Astbury, J. (1980). Labour pain: the role of childbirth education, information and expectation. In *Problems in pain* (C. Peck and M. Wallace, eds). London: Pergamon.

Balaskas, J. (1994). *Preparing for Birth with Yoga*. Dorset: Element Books.

Bonica, J. J. (1975). The nature of pain of parturition. In *Obstetric analgesia and anaesthesia: recent advances and current status* (J. J. Bonica, ed.). New York: Saunders Company.

Bonica, J. J. (1984). Pain research and therapy: recent advances and future needs. In *Advances in Pain Research and Therapy (Vol. 6), Neural Mechanisms of Pain* (L. Kruger and J. Liebeskind, eds). New York: Raven Press.

Bonica, J. J. and Akamatsu, T. (1975). Current concepts of pain of labour and parturition. In *Obstetric analgesia and anaesthesia: recent advances and current status* (J. J. Bonica, ed.). New York: Saunders Company.

Cervero, F. (1994). Sensory innervation of the viscera: peripheral basis of visceral pain. *Physiological Reviews*, **74**, 95–138.

Cogan, R. and Spinnato, J. A. (1986). Pain and discomfort thresholds in late pregnancy. *Pain*, **27**, 63–8.

Copstick, S., Taylor, K., Hayes, R. and Morris, N. (1986). Partner support and use of coping techniques in labour. *Journal of Psychosomatic Research*, **30**, 497–503.

Cosminsky, S. (1977). Childbirth and Midwifery on a Guatemalan Finca. *Medical Anthropology*, **1**, 69–101.

Crawford, J. S. (1972). The second thousand epidural blocks in an obstetric hospital practice. *British Journal of Anaesthetics*, **44**, 1277.

Curry, P., Pascoo, C. and Heap, D. (1994). Patient-controlled epidural in obstetric anaesthetic practice. *Pain*, **57**, 125–8.

Dick Read, G. (1933). *Natural childbirth.* London: Heinemann.

Dick Read, G. (1947). *Revelations of childbirth.* London: Heinemann.

Drewett, R., Kahn, H., Parkhurst, S. and Whiteley, S. (1987). Pain during breastfeeding: the first three months postpartum. *Journal of Reproductive Psychology*, **5**, 183–6.

Dunbar, A. H., Price, D. D. and Newton, R. A. (1988). An assessment of pain responses to thermal stimuli during stages of pregnancy. *Pain*, **35**, 265–9.

Eisenach, J. C., Dobson, C. E., Inturrisi, C., Hood, D. D. and Agner, P. B. (1990). Effect of pregnancy and pain on cerebrospinal fluid immunoreactive enkephalins and norepinephrine in healthy humans. *Pain*, **43**, 149–54.

Folkman, S. (1984). Personal control and stress and coping processes: a theoretical analysis. *Journal of Personality and Social Psychology*, **45**, 829–52.

Fridth, G., Kopare, T., Gaston-Johansson, F. and Norvell, K. T. (1988). Factors associated with more intense labor pain. *Research in Nursing and Health*, **11**, 117–24.

Gaston-Johansson, F., Fridth, G. and Turner-Norvell, K. T. (1988). Progression of labor pain in primiparas and multiparas. *Nursing Research*, **37**, 86–90.

Gijsbers, K. and McGrew, W. C. (1985). Painful birth in non-human primates? Comment on Lefebvre and Carli. *Pain*, **18**, 257.

Gijsbers, K. and Niven, C. (1993). Women and the experience of pain. In *The Health Psychology of Women* (C. Niven and D. Carroll, eds). Switzerland: Harwood Academic Publishers.

Gintzler, A. (1980). Endorphin mediated increases in pain threshold during pregnancy. *Science*, **210**, 193–5.

Goolkasian, P. and Rimer, B. (1984). Pain reactions in pregnant women. *Pain*, **20**, 87–95.

Hapidou, E. G. and DeCatanzaro, D. (1992). Responsiveness to laboratory pain in women as a function of age and childbirth experience. *Pain*, **48**, 177–81.

Harkness, J. and Gijsbers, K. (1989). Pain and stress during childbirth and time of day. *Ethology and Sociobiology*, **10**, 255–61.

Harrison, A. (1991). Childbirth in Kuwait: the experiences of three groups of Arab mothers. *Journal of Pain and Sympton Management*, **6**, 466–75.

Hosobuchi, Y., Adams, J. E. and Linchitz, R. (1977). Pain relief by electrical stimulation of the central gray matter in humans. *Science*, **177**, 183–6.

Illingworth, R. S., Stone, D. G. H. (1952). Self-demand feeding in a maternity unit. *Lancet*, **1**, 682.

Johnson, J. E., Rice, V. A., Fullar, E. S. and Endress, M. P. (1978). Sensory information, instruction in a coping strategy and recovery from surgery. *Research in Nursing and Health*, **1**, 4–17.

Jordan, B. (1980). *Birth in Four Cultures: A cross cultural investigation of childbirth in Yucatan, Holland, Sweden and the United States.* Montreal: Eden Press Women's Publishers.

Kennel, J. H., Klaus, M. J., McGrath, S. (1988). Medical intervention: the effect of social support in labor. *Journal of Paediatric Research*, **5**, 28–31.

Kitzinger, S. (1989). Perceptions of pain in home and hospital deliveries. In *The Free Woman: women's health in the 1990s* (E. V. van Hall and W. Everaerd, eds). Lancashire: Parthenon.

Larsson, P-G., Platz-Christensen, J-J., Bergman, B. and Wallstersson, G. (1991). Advantage or disadvantage of episiotomy compared with spontaneous perineal laceration. *Gynecological Obstetric Investigations*, **31**, 213–16.

Linburg, D. (1982). Primate obstetrics: the biology of birth. *American Journal of Primatology*, Supplement 1, 193–99.

Lowe, N. K. (1989). Explaining the pain of active labor: the importance of maternal confidence. *Research in Nursing and Health*, **12**, 237–45.

MacArthur, C., Lewis, M. and Knox, E. (1992). Investigation of long term problems after obstetric epidural anaesthesia. *British Medical Journal*, **304**, 1279–82.

McIntosh, J. (1989). Models of childbirth and social class: a study of 80 working class primi-gravidae. In *Midwives, Research and Childbirth. Volume 1* (S. Robinson and A. M. Thomson, eds). London: Chapman and Hall.

Marx, J. L. (1979). Dysmenorrhoea: basic research leads to rational theory. *Science*, **205**, 175–6.

Melzack, R. (1975). The McGill Pain Questionnaire: major properties and scoring methods. *Pain*, **1**, 277–99.

Melzack, R. (1984). The myth of painless childbirth. *Pain*, **19**, 321–7.

Melzack, R. and Belanger, E. (1989). Labour pain: correlations with menstrual pain and acute low-back pain before and during pregnancy. *Pain*, **36**, 225–9.

Melzack, R., Belanger, E. and Lacroix, R. (1991). Labor pain: effect of maternal position on front and back pain. *Journal of Pain and Symptom Management*, **6**, 476–80.

Melzack, R., Taenzer, P., Feldman, P. and Kinch, R. A. (1981). Labour is still painful after prepared childbirth training. *Canadian Medical Association Journal*, **125**, 357–63.

Melzack, R. and Wall, P. D. (1993). *The Challenge of Pain*. Harmondsworth: Penguin.

Morgan, B., Bulpitt, C. J., Clifton, P. and Lewis, P. J. (1982). Analgesia and satisfaction in childbirth (the Queen Charlotte's 1,000 mother survey). *Lancet*, **2**, 808–10.

Morse, J. M. (1989). Cultural variation in behavioural response to parturition: Childbirth in Fiji. *Medical Anthropology*, **12**, 35–54.

Nelson, M. K. (1983). Working class women, middle class women and models of childbirth. *Social Problems*, **30** (3), 284–7.

Niven, C. (1986). Factors Affecting Labour Pain. Unpublished doctoral thesis. University of Stirling.

Niven, C. (1992). *Psychological care for Families: before, during and after birth*. Oxford: Butterworth-Heinemann.

Niven, C. (1994). Coping with labour pain: the midwife's role. In *Midwives, Research and Childbirth. Volume 3* (S. Robinson and A. Thomson, eds). London: Chapman and Hall.

Niven, C. and Gijsbers, K. (1984). Obstetric and non-obstetric factors related to labour pain. *Journal of Reproductive and Infant Psychology*, **2**, 61–78.

Niven, C. and Gijsbers, K. (1989). Do low levels of labour pain reflect low sensitivity to noxious stimulation? *Social Science and Medicine*, **29**, 585–8.

Niven, C. and Gijsbers, K. (in press). Coping with labour pain.

Norvell, K. T., Gaston-Johansson, F. and Fridh, G. (1988). Remembrance of labor pain: how valid are retrospective measurements? *Pain*, **31**, 77–86.

Paech, M. (1992). Patient controlled analgesia in labour – is continuous infusion of benefit? *Anaesthesia and Intensive Care*, **20**, 15–20.

Purdie, J., Reid, J., Thorburn, J. and Asbury, A. (1992). Continuous extradural analgesia: comparison of midwife top-ups, continuous infusions and patient controlled administration. *British Journal of Anaesthesia*, **68**, 580–84.

Reading, A. (1982). How women view post-episiotomy pain. *British Medical Journal*, **284**, 283.

Robson, K. and Kumar, R. (1981). Maternal sexuality. *British Journal of Obstetrics and Gynaecology*, **88**, 882.

Rushton, E. and McGrew, W. C. (1980). Breech birth of a chimpanzee (*Pan Troglodytes*). *Journal of Medical Primatology*, **9**, 183–93.

Scott-Palmer, J. and Skevington, S. (1981). Pain during childbirth and menstruation: a study of locus of control. *Journal of Psychosomatic Research*, **3**, 151–5.

Skovlund, E., Fyllingen, G., Landre, H. and Nesheim, B.-I. (1991). Comparison of postpartum pain treatments using a sequential trial design: 11. Naproxen versus paracetamol. *European Journal of Clinical Pharmacology*, **40**, 539–42.

Slade, P., MacPherson, S. A., Hume, A. and Maresh, M. (1993). Expectation, experiences and satisfaction with labour. *British Journal of Clinical Psychology*, **32**, 469–83.

Steinman, J. L., Komisaruk, B. R., Yaksh, T. L. and Tyce, G. M. (1983). Spinal cord monoamines modulate the antinociceptive effects of vaginal stimulation in rats. *Pain*, **16**, 155–66.

Stewart, D. E. (1982). Psychiatric symptoms following attempted natural childbirth. *Canadian Medical Association Journal*, **127**, 713–16.

Thacker, S. and Banta, H. (1983). Benefits and risks of episiotomy: an interpretive review of the English language literature, 1860–1980. *Obstetrical and Gynecological Survey*, **38**, 322–38.

Whipple, B. and Komisaruk, B. R. (1985). Elevation of pain threshold by vaginal stimulation in women. *Pain*, **21**, 357–67.

Whipple, B., Josimovich, J. B. and Komisaruk, B. R. (1990). Sensory thresholds during the antepartum, intrapartum and post partum periods. *International Journal of Nursing Studies*, **27**, 213–21.

Wolkind, S. and Zajicek, E. (1981). *Pregnancy: a psychological and social study*. London: Academic Press.

12

Stillbirth and neonatal death

Jane Littlewood

> This is a sad but extremely important final chapter, sensitively written by Jane
> Littlewood. It reminds us that conception, birth and death are all parts of the
> essential process of transition between existence and non-existence. In it Jane
> shows how inappropriate care can add to the intrinsic suffering caused by the loss
> of a baby at birth or while in a neonatal unit. She addresses the theoretical issues
> raised by the loss of a baby with whom the parents have had little contact, in
> circumstances which are highly traumatic. In this way this chapter is closely
> related to the contents of Chapter 6 on miscarriage.
>
> By raising the issue of babies in neonatal care, this chapter also provides a link
> forward to a chapter in Volume 3 in this series which will deal with premature
> babies in neonatal units.

Introduction

Whilst this chapter is primarily concerned with stillbirth and neonatal death it
begins with a consideration of the ways in which stillbirth and neonatal deaths
were routinely handled prior to recent policy and practice changes in the United
Kingdom. The chapter continues with a discussion of the process of grief itself
and of the factors which are widely believed to complicate this process. It will
be shown that the death of a baby is highly likely to be associated with
complications arising during the process of grief. However, it will also be shown
that good professional practice, at and around the time of the death, may go some
way to minimizing the possibility of such complications.

The particular impact of stillbirths, both expected and unexpected, will be
considered and a discussion of circumstances surrounding the deaths of babies
in neonatal units is also included. The impact of the death of a baby on future
childbearing will be discussed and the chapter concludes by identifying the
relevant areas for, and importance of, future research concerning stillbirth and
neonatal death.

Rugby-tackle management

Up until approximately 15 years ago the death of a baby at, or around the time
of, birth was subject to what has been termed 'rugby-tackle management'
(Mander, 1994). According to Mander, 'rugby-tackle management' involved a
combination of the following five courses of action:

1. Remove the dead body from the room as quickly as possible (hence the term
   rugby-tackle management, to emphasize the speed and method by which this
   manoeuvre was achieved).

2. Discourage the parents from seeing the baby.
3. Discourage the parents from communicating about the baby.
4. Encourage the parents to forget about the loss and to concentrate upon conceiving another baby.
5. Institutional disposal of the baby's body – often in an unmarked mass grave.

The full impact of such well-meaning but misguided attempts at management were often long term. For example:

> My mother took him and wrapped him in his shawl. She had him, she was the other side of the bedroom door with him and the doctor wouldn't let her in. He said it was better if I didn't see him. I'll regret that until the day I die. I couldn't have any more you see and I never even saw him. My mother said he was beautiful.
>
> Littlewood, 1992b

This particular comment was made by a woman during an interview concerning her husband's death. She was 84 years old and her baby had died 60 years prior to her comments.

In one of the relatively early arguments for changing professional practice Lewis (1979) summarized the impact of such practice in the following way:

> This avoidance by the helping professionals extends into the neglect of the study of the effect of stillbirth on the mother and the family. There is a conspiracy of silence. We seem unwilling to come to terms with the fact that it is a tragedy which can seriously affect the mental health of the bereaved mother and her family. After the failure to mourn, mothers can have psychotic breakdowns or there can be severe mental difficulties. Children born before or after a stillbirth where there has been a failure to mourn a stillbirth can have severe emotional difficulties.

However, Morris (1988) showed how, in less than a decade, practice had radically changed in some areas:

> The routine photography of all stillborn and now even miscarriages and practices such as giving parents the baby's name tag, lock of hair or other memento shows how much progress has been made.

Changes in professional practice were supported by self-help initiatives developed by parents. In 1992, the SANDS (Stillbirth and Neonatal Death Society) guidelines were given official endorsement in England and Wales by a central government committee. Specifically:

> We recommended that the guidelines drawn up for SANDS should form the basis for training of all professionals and managers involved in maternity care for dealing with bereavement. All units should ensure that such training is given to staff in a properly designed way.
>
> HMSO, 1992

The committee's overall conclusions are also of interest:

> We conclude that the evidence highlighted the overarching need for professionals to take account of best practice in this area and to formulate

coherent and sensitive policies to address the needs of parents and families who experience miscarriage, stillbirth and neonatal death.

HMSO, 1992

Essentially this adoption of the SANDS guidelines represented a reversal of the previous mode of 'management'. Far from being encouraged to forget, parents are now encouraged to remember their baby. Mementos are made available and parents are encouraged to talk openly about their loss. Furthermore, parents frequently view the body of their baby and dispose of the body with ritual. However, the death of a child, at or around the time of birth, remains a profoundly painful experience and best practice may not always be taken into account. For example:

> I was left holding Hester while people, as it seemed to me, backed off into the corners of the room. I spoke to her and cried with her ... I held out my hand towards the retreating figures and asked for help. They retreated further and further away.

Fairbairn, 1992

Whilst the avoidance of both people who are dying and their relatives is an extremely common experience reported by people who have been bereaved (Littlewood, 1992a) this particular example of it had unfortunate consequences for the father in question because eventually, in a state of confusion and considerable emotional distress, he left his baby to be with his wife and retrospectively; '... wondered what possessed me to let my baby die in a room full of strangers while I ran off and hid from her'.

Obviously, whilst the adoption of good practice by health care professionals is to be advocated, it can be argued that the loss of a baby in contemporary society is one of the most difficult bereavements to cope with and, as such, will inevitably be associated with high levels of parental distress. The following section of the chapter identifies, in general, why this should be the case.

The process of grief in contemporary western society

The process of grieving amongst the general adult population has been relatively well documented by numerous researchers and it is possible, despite the wide variation in individual experiences, to identify a very general pattern associated with uncomplicated grief (Littlewood, 1992a). The initial response following the death of a loved person is usually one of shock and disbelief. However, despite an apparent inability to comprehend the loss the person may suffer from outbursts of intense emotion, for example, panic, sobbing or irrational anger.

The person goes on to experience an intense physical, emotional and cognitive reaction to the loss. The bereaved person longs for the return of the dead person and appears to be completely preoccupied by his/her image. Events immediately preceding the death are obsessively reviewed in an often abortive attempt to understand what has happened. Self-reproach for having caused, or failed to prevent, the death is often present and anger, directed at the self or others is a frequently cited component of grief. Dreams and vivid hallucinations may occur and a period of social withdrawal frequently accompanies this intense preoccupation with the dead person.

Following, or interspersed with, these experiences are feelings of apathy, fatigue and despair. Difficulty in concentration and disrupted sleeping patterns are commonly reported and thoughts of suicide are sometimes present. Eventually, episodes of relative normality occur for progressively longer periods of time and episodes of grief decrease in frequency. The general consensus of researchers in the area would indicate that the whole process may take up to two years to progress to a point where 'pangs' of grief are relatively self-contained and occasional episodes. However, Raphael (1984) indicates that the deaths of children in general are often associated with what she calls 'shadow grief' in which the parents project the dead child's expected developmental path into the future and experience pangs of grief at, for example, the time when the dead child would have been expected to start school.

Descriptions of complicated grief are not uncommon and these descriptions may be loosely gathered under three headings: delayed grief, chronic grief and absent or distorted grief. Delayed grief occurs when the recognition of the loss is postponed. Typically grief is experienced with particular severity at a later date. Chronic grief is associated with instances in which the expected range of reactions are present but the bereaved person does not recover from them. Raphael (1984) has suggested that in distorted reactions to bereavement one aspect of grief is emphasized and others often suppressed. She further suggests that the two common patterns are extreme expressions of either anger or guilt. The apparent absence of grief has also been noted and Bowlby (1969) has suggested that whilst grief may be absent other bereavement-related problems are usually present.

Whilst there have been many researchers who have documented complications which may arise during the process of grieving, Worden (1992) usefully groups the relevant risk factors under five headings: relational, historical, circumstantial, personality and social.

Unfortunately, the death of a baby is associated with difficulties relevant to at least three of these headings: the relational, the circumstantial and the social.

Specifically, narcissistic relationships in which the decreased represents an extension of the self have been found by Worden (1992) to be associated with complications arising during the grieving process. Furthermore, the likely circumstances surrounding the death of a baby, i.e. the uncertainty (Lazare, 1979), the absence of a body (Simpson, 1979) and the unanticipated and untimely nature of the death (Parkes, 1972) have all been associated with complicated grief. Finally, losses which are socially unspeakable or socially negated (Lazare, 1979) and the absence of a social support network (Vachon, Sheldon, Lancee, et al., 1982) have also been identified as contributing to complications arising during the process of grief. To a greater or lesser extent, all of these problems are associated with the death of a baby.

Bereavement at the time of childbirth

The very nature of the relationship between parents and babies who die make the nature of the loss more difficult to cope with. Raphael (1984) suggests that parents commit themselves to a baby in the hope that the baby will eventually gratify their own unfulfilled hopes and dreams. Thus the baby may come to represent not only a physical but a psychological extension of the parents (Rando, 1986). These 'narcissistic' expectations are obviously dashed if the baby should die and the mother may be left grieving not only for a baby but for a part of herself which may be seen to be indistinguishable from her child (Peretz, 1970).

Furthermore, Borg and Lasker (1982) suggest that the sheer intensity of the mother's feelings of grief may induce fear in the mother because the strength of her feelings do not match any tangible contact with the baby. Consequently, it is often difficult for the mother to understand exactly why she is so upset over a baby she barely knew. However, it is not only the intensity of feelings of grief but the sheer complexity of them which may cause difficulties. Hutchins (1986) summarizes these difficulties in terms of trying to say 'hello and goodbye' at the same time. This difficulty may account for some parental experiences of temporary 'euphoria' following seeing the body of their baby.

For example, a father described ordering flowers for the funeral, immediately after viewing his daughter's body in the following way:

> I don't know if what happened in the florists can be explained or not but it was very unusual. We walked in feeling on air ... we were laughing and joking ... and generally gave the impression that we were ordering flowers for a party rather than a funeral.

Littlewood, 1992b

As Nichols (1984) points out, the very intimacy of the parents' relationship to their baby makes the loss difficult to talk about – the hopes and dreams were essentially personal ones and may not be easy to either identify or share with other people.

Lewis and Bourne (1989) attribute maternal difficulty in accepting the loss of a baby to the uncertain and bewildering circumstances in which the death occurs, the mother may 'half know' of the death but can scarcely, due to the unexpected nature of the event, bring herself to believe it. Lewis and Bourne liken the situation to that following 'missing, presumed dead' verdicts – situations in which complicated grief frequently occurs (Lazare, 1979). For example:

> They'd told me he was dead but I just didn't believe it. The midwife said that I could have strong pain relief during labour because nothing I did would hurt the baby. I didn't have any pain relief, I wanted it to hurt because I thought that if it hurt he would be all right. When he was born, all I can remember thinking was please, please, don't let him be dead.

Littlewood, 1992a

The death of a baby is clearly both unexpected and untimely and both of these factors have been associated with complicated grief (Parkes, 1972). Kellner and Lake (1986) suggest that this exacerbates maternal feelings of confusion and loss of control. Mander (1994) indicates that 'survivor guilt' may be present and feelings concerning 'it should have been me' further increase the woman's distress and confusion.

Lack of tangible memories may also leave a woman wondering why she is experiencing grief. Obviously, the adoption of the SANDS guidelines go some way to minimizing these circumstantial factors which are now well documented as being distressing and confusing. However, another circumstantial factor which affects the process of grief is age. A woman who bears children is usually young and in contemporary society young people are rarely confronted by death or grief (Littlewood, 1992a). Consequently, young people find these issues particularly difficult to cope with. Cooper (1980) points out that young parents tend to respond with anger and outrage over the death of a baby and these responses are thought to bode ill in respect of the grieving process (Raphael, 1984).

Social support also proves difficult following the death of a baby. At one level the meaning of the pregnancy is unique to the mother and, to a greater or lesser extent the father, but the meaning of such a loss is essentially hidden from others and the mother may feel particularly isolated (Lewis and Bourne, 1989; Rando, 1986).

In terms of the wider society, the relatively infrequent deaths of babies are shrouded in secrecy (Borg and Lasker, 1982). Consequently, the mother may feel irrationally ashamed about her loss and be unwilling to speak about it. Furthermore, since the baby's death occurred in hospital, many people in the general community may treat the baby as a 'non-person' and trivialize the loss (Nichols, 1984). In an early piece of work, Bourne (1968) showed that GPs were extremely reluctant to even remember anything about a woman who had experienced a stillbirth – again, this type of avoidance has been shown to further complicate the process of grieving amongst the general population (Lazare, 1979).

Overall, the elements of lack of anticipation, difficulty in accepting the loss and lack of social support would all seem to combine to make the death of a baby uniquely difficult to cope with.

Stillbirth

Stillbirth is, mercifully, a rare occurrence. However, when it does occur, what is expected to be a joyful event turns into a tragedy which is typically unexpected by the mother and those in attendance. Kirkley-Best and Kellner (1982), in their review of the area, indicate that the commonest circumstances surrounding still-birth are those in which the baby is viable until labour. Even in cases where there is forewarning of the death, these authors suggest that this may be met with a lack of comprehension on the part of the parents. Consequently, parental reaction to the occurrence of a stillbirth may be similar in both instances.

Whilst in general circumstances, a period of time in which to anticipate that a death will occur has been argued to be beneficial to those about to be bereaved, Jolly (1987) suggests that the mother carrying a dead baby may feel like a 'living coffin'. Alternatively, Hutchins (1986) argues that the mother may beneficially begin anticipatory grief in the antenatal period but, as Grubb (1976) and Kish (1978) point out, the situation is complicated because profound disturbances of body image featuring uncleanliness and horror may be present.

For various reasons, some medical and some psychological, the induction of labour is usually recommended in these cases and Dyer (1992) suggests that waiting for a day or two may better enable the mother to orientate herself to the loss but, whilst more research clearly needs to be conducted in this area, the overall evidence would indicate that the woman may persist in 'hoping for the best'. Furthermore, Mander (1994) indicates that the mother may not be alone with her hopes. Specifically:

> There is a moment at the birth when everyone who is present, the parents and the staff, see that the baby has been born and hope against hope that the baby is going to cry. I know that it's quite illogical, but you still hope. And it is not until that moment when we all realise that the baby really is dead, that we all finally realise it is so.

In cases of unexpected stillbirth, shock remains the primary feature (Hutchins, 1986) and initial reactions appear to be minimal (Bourne, 1968). However, Wolff, Nielson and Schiller (1970) noted a tendency towards anger for up to three years after the event. These researchers also noted a tendency for parents to either seek solace in another child or to develop a fear of pregnancy and child-birth. Culberg (1971) conducted a similar study and found that approximately one-third of mothers were experiencing symptoms which were severe enough to warrant the diagnosis of a psychiatric illness.

Alternatively, Cooper (1980) indicated that the couples in her study perceived the stillbirth as a threat to their integrity or a medical accident to be exposed rather than as a loss to be mourned. In this sense, the reactions would appear to be similar to the reactions of parents who have lost children in disasters. As Hodgkinson (1989) has indicated:

> Following the Zeebrugge disaster, parents who had lost adult children, for whom no compensation was indicated in British law, banded together to form the Herald Families Association. They were enraged that they were symbolically denied recognition that they had been bereaved. Their avowed aim was to see the prosecution of the ferry operator for negligence and the institution of safer ferry standards. It remains to be seen whether this channelling of anger will prove an aid or a block to resolution.

Whilst there is an urgent need for more research in the area of long-term adjustment to stillbirth, it seems reasonable to suggest that the factors surrounding stillbirth may make the process of grief painfully difficult and complicated.

Neonatal death

Babies are admitted to neonatal units (NNU) when a health problem has either been recognized or is likely to arise. Loss is a predominant theme amongst the parents of such babies irrespective of whether or not their baby dies. The ideal baby they expected to have is lost (Sherr, 1989) and the anticipated role of primary care-giver has been lost too (Kennell, Slyler and Klaus, 1970). Furthermore, the specialist and highly technical nature of the care given in NNUs has been shown to make mothers feel both incompetent and superfluous in terms of their perception of their abilities to care for their babies (Breen, 1978).

Benfield, Leib and Volman (1978) argue that grieving a baby who has died in an NNU is a highly individual experience but that parental concerns include anger, guilt, disbelief and a sense of unreality. Whilst grief is never easy Lewis and Bourne (1989) have suggested that neonatal death is not so shocking as still-birth because the parents have had time to be with their baby and therefore find it easier to attribute personhood to him or her. Furthermore, the presence of the staff in the NNU, who have all been committed to the care of the baby may, to a certain extent, help the parents to validate the social existence of the baby (Littlewood, 1992a).

Alternatively, helplessly watching a futile struggle for survival may serve to sharpen an already deeply felt distress. For example:

> At the birth of her child Ms W felt that if he was going to have to be kept alive artificially, then it was better that he should die. However, when she saw her son he looked better than she expected and efforts were made. By the third day of his life Ms W felt differently and desperately hoped that her son would survive. However, she was told that there was no hope of his recovery and that the machines were to be switched off. Ms W felt that the fact that her son had struggled to survive made his personality seem that much stronger, so the decision to let him die was much harder to take ... Ms W remembered feeling shattered when the death finally occurred.
>
> Littlewood, 1992a

Also, anticipatory loss may lead parents to feel uncertain about forming a relationship with an ill baby (Kennell and Klaus, 1982). This may, paradoxically, result in guilt if the baby subsequently dies.

Furthermore, the tendency for the broader community to avoid or minimize the extent of a loss when a baby dies in an NNU would appear to be comparable to communal reactions, or rather more accurately the lack of them, to a stillbirth (Helmrath and Steinitz, 1978). Nichols (1986) attributes most of the problems encountered by parents of dying newborns to discounted grief and negated death. Again, more research is required in order to clarify these issues.

Future childbearing

Whilst the decision to embark upon another pregnancy following a stillbirth or neonatal death is highly individual (Wolff, Nielson and Schiller, 1970) an urgent desire for another pregnancy at a relatively early stage of grieving is, in itself, believed to further complicate the process of grief. Leon (1990) interprets the prevalence and urgency of such desires in terms of the mother's damaged self-esteem and argues that a subsequent successful pregnancy becomes the only route by which the woman believes she will regain her equilibrium.

However, whilst Lewis and Bourne (1989) agree that a subsequent pregnancy may shorten grief they indicate that the effect is temporary and argue that grief may re-emerge either at the time of the subsequent birth or at some unforeseeable time in the future. Whilst the longer-term implications are difficult to foresee and research, Mander (1994) feels confident enough to assert that, at least in the short term: '... we may be certain that a mother who hurries or is hurried into another pregnancy is likely to find the experience unpleasant or even traumatic'.

However, the desire to have a child may be particularly strong and whilst a subsequent pregnancy may well be indicative of problems associated with grief this may not always be the case. Nevertheless, health care professionals need to be aware of the special needs that a woman who has lost a child and is embarking upon a subsequent pregnancy may have.

Conclusion

This chapter has been concerned with the nature of the grieving process follow-ing stillbirth and neonatal death. It has been suggested that recent changes in practice may, given the generic knowledge concerning the process of grief, go some way to ameliorating parental distress. Contemporary practice should mitigate the sense of unreality and confusion which are inevitably present following the death of a baby. In short, the available evidence would suggest that we no longer, albeit unwittingly, make things worse. However, actual research concerning the impact of the introduction of the SANDS guidelines is long overdue.

The death of a baby is always a tragedy for the parents and the evidence would indicate that the lack of availability of support in the community should give cause for concern since the factors surrounding the death of a child at, or around the time of, birth are precisely those which are known to complicate the process of grief amongst the adult population in general. Stillbirth would appear to be associated with anger and outrage following the death to a greater extent than deaths which occur in an NNU. However, this is another area which would benefit from further research. Alternatively, deaths which occur in NNUs may be associated with ambivalence and guilt which may cause the parents additional distress. Further investigation is needed to clarify these issues.

Despite the fact of the rarity of the loss of a baby in the first few days of life, such a loss represents a potential disaster for the parents. Consequently, we urgently need to further our understanding of the aftermath, in both the short and the long term, of such a loss. Many parents whose baby dies in the first few days of life go on to have other children and the evidence would suggest that they need a great deal of care and support.

Whilst it is customary to point out that all losses carry within them the potential for personal growth, the benefits of grief are not immediately apparent to people who have been bereaved. The circumstances surrounding the death of a baby would appear to indicate that parents will require a great deal of support if this potential is to be realized.

Applications

The following references may be consulted for recommenda-tions for practice:

- SANDS (1991). *Miscarriage, Stillbirth and Neonatal Death, Guidelines for Professionals.* London: SANDS.
- Worden, J. W. (1992). *Grief Counselling and Grief Therapy: A Handbook for the Mental Health Practitioner* (2nd ed.). London: Routledge.

Further reading

Kohner, N. and Henley, A. (1991). *When a baby dies: The experience of late miscarriage stillbirth and neonatal death.* London: Pandora Press.
Leon, I. G. (1990). *When a Baby Dies: Psychotherapy for Pregnancy and Newborn Loss.* London: Yale University Press.
Littlewood, J. (1992). *Aspects of Grief: Bereavement in Adult Life.* London: Routledge.
Mander, R. (1994). *Loss and Bereavement in Childbearing.* London: Blackwell Scientific Publications.
Rando, T. A. (1986). *Parental Loss of a Child.* Champaign, Illinois: Research Press.

References

Benfield, G. Leib, S. and Volman, J. (1978). Grief Response of Parents to Neonatal Death and Parent Participation in Deciding Care. *Paediatrics,* **62,** 171–7.
Bourne, S. (1968). The Psychological Effects of Stillbirth on Women and their Doctors. *Journal of the Royal College of General Practitioners,* **16,** 103–12.
Borg, S. and Lasker, J. (1982). *When Pregnancy Fails.* London: Routledge.
Bowlby, J. (1969). Attachment and Loss, Volume 1. London: Hogarth Press.
Breen, D. (1978). The Mother and the Hospital. In *Tearing the Veil: Essays of Femininity* (S. Lipshitz, ed.). London: Routledge/Kegan Paul.
Cooper, J. D. (1980). Parental Reactions to Stillbirth. *British Journal of Social Work,* **10,** 55–69.
Culburg, J. (1971). Mental Reactions of Women to Perinatal Death, Proceedings of the Third Congress of Psychosomatic Medicine in Obstetrics and Gynaecology, Basel, Karger, Switzerland.
Dyer, M. (1992). Stillborn – Still Precious. *Midwives Information and Resource Service, Midwifery Digest,* **2:** 2, 341–4.
Fairbairn, G. (1992). When a Baby Dies – A Father's View. In *Death, Dying and Bereavement* (D. Dickenson and M. Johnson, eds). London: Sage.
Grubb, C. A. (1976). Body Image Concerns of a Multipara in the Situation of Intrauterine Fetal Death. *Maternal Child Nursing,* **5,** 93.
HMSO (1992). *Health Committee (2nd report) Maternity Services, Vol. 1.* London: HMSO.
Helmrath, T. A. and Steinitz, E. M. (1978). Death of an Infant: Parental Grieving and the Failure of Social Support. In *Parental Loss of a Child* (T. Rando, ed.). Champaign, Illinois: Research Press.
Hodgkinson, P. E. (1989). Technological Disaster – Survival and Bereavement. *Social Science and Medicine,* **55,** 29–34.
Hutchins, S. H. (1986). Stillbirth. In *Parental Loss of a Child* (T. Rando, ed.). Champaign, Illinois: Research Press.
Jolly, J. (1987). *Missed Beginnings.* London: Austen Cornish Publishers.
Kellner, K. R. and Lake, M. (1986). Grief Counselling. In *High Risk Pregnancy* (R. A. Knuppel and J. E. Drukker, eds). Philadelphis: W. B. Saunders.
Kennell, J. H. and Klaus, M. H. (1982). Caring for the Parents of Premature or Sick Infants. In *Parent Infant Bonding* (2nd ed.) (M. H. Klaus and J. H. Kennell, eds). St Louis: Mosby.
Kennell, J., Slyter, H. and Klaus, M. H. (1970). The Mourning Responses of Parents on the Death of a Newborn Infant. *New England Journal of Medicine,* **283,** 344–9.
Kirkley-Best, E. and Kellner, K. (1982). The Forgotten Grief: A Review of the Psychology of Stillbirth. *American Journal of Orthopsychiatry,* **52,** 420–9.
Kish, G. (1978). Notes on C. Grubb's Body Image Concerns of a Multipara in the Situation of Intrauterine Fetal Death. *Maternal Child Nursing Journal,* **7,** 11.
Kohner, N. and Henley, A. (1991). *When a baby dies: The experience of late miscarriage stillbirth and neonatal death.* London: Pandora Press.
Lazare, A. (1979). Unresolved Grief. In *Outpatient Psychiatry: Diagnosis and Treatment* (A. Lazare, ed.). Baltimore: Williams and Wilkins.

Leon, I. G. (1990). *When a Baby Dies: Psychotherapy for Pregnancy and Newborn Loss.* London: Yale University Press.

Lewis, E. (1979). Mourning by the Family after a Stillbirth or Neonatal Death. *Archives of Disease in Childhood,* **55**, 303–6.

Lewis, E. and Bourne, S. (1989). Perinatal Death. In *Psychological Aspects of Obstetrics and Gynaecology* (M. Oates, ed.). London: Bailliere Tindall.

Littlewood, J. (1992a). Aspects of Grief: Bereavement in Adult Life. London: Routledge.

Littlewood, J. (1992b). A Comparison of Maternal Experiences of Stillbirth and Neonatal Death. Unpublished paper presented to the Annual Conference of the Society for Reproductive and Infant Psychology, Glasgow, Sept.

Mander, R. (1994). *Loss and Bereavement in Childbearing.* London: Blackwell Scientific Publications.

Morris, D. (1988). Management of Perinatal Bereavement. *Archives of Disease in Childhood,* **63**, 870–72.

Nichols, J. A. (1984). Illegitimate Mourners. In *Children and Death: Perspectives and Challenges Symposium.* Akron, Ohio.

Nichols, J. A. (1986). Newborn Death. In Parental Loss of a Child (T. Rando, ed.). Champaign, Illinois: Research Press.

Parkes, C. M. (1972). *Bereavement.* New York: International Universities Press.

Peretz, D. (1970). Reactions to Loss. In *Loss and Grief: Psychological Management in Medical Practice* (B. Schoenberg, D. Karr, D. Peretz and A. H. Kutsher, eds). Columbia: Columbia University Press.

Rando, T. A. (ed.) (1986). *Parental Loss of a Child.* Champaign, Illinois: Research Press.

Raphael, B. (1984). *The Anatomy of Bereavement: A Handbook for the Caring Professions.* London: Unwin Hyman.

SANDS (1991). *Miscarriage, Stillbirth and Neonatal Death, Guidelines for Professionals.* London: SANDS.

Sherr, L. (ed.) (1989). *Death, Dying and Bereavement.* Oxford: Blackwell Scientific Publications.

Simpson, M. A. (1979). *The Facts of Death.* Englewood Cliffs, NJ: Prentice-Hall.

Vachon, M. L. S., Sheldon, A. R., Lancee, S. L., Lyall, W. A. L., Roger, J. and Freeman, S. J. (1982). Correlates of Enduring Distress Following Bereavement: Social Network Life Situation and Personality. *Psychological Medicine,* **12**, 783–8.

Wolff, J. R., Nielson, P. E. and Schiller, P. (1970). The Emotional Reaction to a Stillbirth. *American Journal of Obstetrics and Gynaecology,* **108**, 73–7.

Worden, J. W. (1992). *Grief Counselling and Grief Therapy: A Handbook for the Mental Health Practitioner* (2nd ed.). London: Routledge.

Index